Gabriel's Dragon

The Author wishes to acknowledge, with special thanks, the unstinting personal and financial support received from the Friends of the Cedars Cancer Institute of the McGill University Health Center. Donations to either Cedars or St. George Antiochian Church are encouraged in exchange for a copy of this publication.

Cedars Cancer Institute of the MUHC
687 Pine Ave., W
Montreal, Canada
H3G 1A1

St George Antiochian Orthodox Church
555 rue Jean Talon est
Montreal, Canada
H2R 1T8

www.cedars.ca

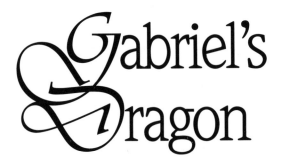

Gabriel's Dragon

ANTONY GABRIEL

Abbeyfield Publishers
2003, Toronto, Canada

Published in 2003 by Abbeyfield Publishers,
a division of The Abbeyfield Companies Ltd.
Suite 103, One Benvenuto Place
Toronto Ontario Canada M4V 2L1
Telephone: 416-925-6458 Fax: 416-925-4165 • E-mail <abbeyfld@istar.ca>

Ordering information
Hushion House
c/o Georgetown Terminal Warehouses
34 Armstrong Avenue, Georgetown ON, L7G 4R9
Tel: 866-485-5556   Fax: 866-485-6665
e-mail: bsisnett@gtwcanada.com

National Library of Canada Cataloguing in Publication

Gabriel, Antony, 1940–
Gabriel's dragon / Antony Gabriel.

Includes bibliographical references.
ISBN 1-894584-12-0 (soft cover)
ISBN 1-894584-16-3 (hard cover)

1. Gabriel, Antony, 1940–. 2. Syrian Orthodox Church—Quebec (Province)—
Montréal—Biography. I. Title.

BX743.9.G32A3 2003   281'.63'092   C2003-900565-8

Book management: Bill Belfontaine
Cover / Interior Design: Karen Petherick,
                    Intuitive Design International Ltd., Ontario, Canada
Cover illustration: Michael Petherick
Back cover photograph: MariLou Bassett
Text fonts: Janson, Vivaldi

Printed and Bound in Canada

Dedication

An extremely precious and precocious nine-year-old was taken from us in July,1997. She is Janna Sarah Lynch. Named after her two great-grandmothers, she is our second eldest grandchild. An untimely automobile accident was the cause of her death after a week in a pediatric trauma unit in Westchester County, New York. A beautiful flower who blossomed briefly in the garden of our lives, she continues her journey to our Father's eternal vale. We speak of Janna always in the present, for although she is in another place outside our time, she lives there and remains alive in our hearts. To this day and forevermore, a tear-filled smile at the mere mention of her name recalls her sweet presence among us. We dedicate this book to her.

Acknowledgements

I wish to thank my beloved wife, Lynn for her long-suffering and tenacity pushing me on ... and for editing my lengthy diary into a readable text, and also acknowledge Christina Richardson who transcribed my personal diary.

My appreciation is also extended to Karen Petherick of Intuitive Design International Ltd., for the unique cover and professional appearance of the pages, and to Bill Belfontaine, my publisher for his encouragement and guidance in publishing this work.

Contents

Page   **Chapter**

ix   Poem – Swirling in the Vortex
xiii   Foreword

1 . . . One   The Nightmare Begins
9 . . . *Poem*   *I call upon You, O God, my mercy*
10 . . . Two   Surgery
23 . . . *Poem*   *Thou hast made us for Thyself*
24 . . . Three   Visions from the Past
38 . . . *Poem*   *I know Lord that you are all powerful*
39 . . . Four   The Questioning Begins
44 . . . *Poem*   *But love whose cause is God*
45 . . . Five   Reflections on a Priestly Life
53 . . . *Poem*   *I will extol You, O Lord (Psalms 30)*
54 . . . Six   The Decision
63 . . . Seven   The Descent
79 . . . *Poem*   *Love is a great thing*
80 . . . Eight   Out of Control
89 . . . *Poem*   *So every faithful heart shall pray (Psalms 32)*
90 . . . Nine   The Turning Point
94 . . . *Poem*   *There is a love like a small lamp*
95 . . . Ten   Celebration, Faith and Community
102 . . . Eleven The Enigma of Life
109 . . . Twelve The Struggle Between Life and Death
123 . . . Thirteen Picking Up the Pieces
132 . . . Fourteen New Beginnings and a Sabbatical
140 . . . Fifteen A Return to Reality
152 . . . *Poem* *A Prayer*

. . . continued

Contents

Page   **Chapter**

153 . . . Sixteen   Onward

156 . . . Seventeen End Point, Beginning Point

160 . . . *Poem*   *Prayer of The Acceptance of God's Will*

161 . . . Epilogue   In the Lion's Den

167 . . . Fini   I Was Asked to Write a Sketch

169 . . . Message From the Publisher

171 . . . End Notes

173 . . . Other Readings

Swirling into the Vortex

— Antony Gabriel

"… My eyes seep sorrow
        water skins with holes"
                Abid bin Al Abras.

Illness, a time of grace: affording one
        the space to reflect,
                forgive the past
                        and move forward to the future.

"Why me" is not the real question; but why NOT
        me? Who am I to be exempted
                from suffering?

Suffering is that creative moment
        of rebirth … the purging of soul's labyrinth
                Can one truly know life's secrets
                        extraneous from
                                the crucible of fire?

In that one moment, everything changes:
        the old walls collapse
                new trenches are forged.

Who can dare prophecize the future
        and what it will bear:
                Oh Pensive One …

Days are eaten up by one another in the
        euphoria of pharmaceutical floating …

Suddenly there is the realization that
                there has been a bridge crossed
        never to return to the land of yesterday …

Life so sweet, so bitter, laughter, tears
　　　commingle together
　　　　　in life's brew.

Presence, strange, mystical; touching, caressing
　　　healing — from the land
　　　　　beyond all other countries.

Yes, Lord. Thy will be done. Or is it
　　　life's endless rhythm?
　　　　　Surrender.

Why? Blame? Or the gestation
　　　bursting with the seeds
　　　　　of sensitivity.

Or the furnace refining;
　　　　　smoothing
　　　making finer
　　　　　interior jewel.

Family, friends those sacred bonds,
　　　the balm that envelopes
　　　　　and binds wounds.

Night, endless night: Oh night, when
　　　will the dawn beckon us
　　　　　to a new day.

Communion; Quiet Presence of that
　　　special someone …
　　　　　Blessing.

Dreams that stir the subconscience,
　　　sleep sweetly interrupted
　　　　　with that Face …
Bread given …　　　Fragrant myrrh.

Antony Gabriel

The grand YES, to the Cross, forever
transforming in the twinkling
of an eye ...
ego lost.

Clarity as never before;
Preciousness of eternity
time, life.

Will anything be the same:
Ever?   Ever?
O heart's agony ...

Endless LOVE burn Thyself
within the bowels
of my heart.

The kingdom so near; distant
calling ...
Fleeting thoughts of pain; unfinished business,
sighs; Ah!
Letting go; forgiveness. A new light.
Yes, new beginnings ...
Suddenly nature opens up its tender embrace.
How did I not notice
snowy mountains,
bright sunrises?

Alleluia! Amen! Hymns. Heaven's elevation
swallowed up
into divinity.

Bodily functions, primitive and essential —
cessation; stirrings
and stumbles.

GABRIEL'S DRAGON

Small laughter at first steps;
the soothing touch of that healer
in whose face one confronts
awakening from the deep.

Tormented insomnia is released
by the pulsating energy
of grace upon grace …

Hosanna: The Ultimate *YES*
to Him …
Oh, Mother Divine
understanding and
conveying our plea
before The Son.

The dark night gradually unfolding
to a new today.
Oh, Compassionate One …
Silence, Stillness,
Centering.

Abandonment into His Arms.
Uplifted.
Yes!

"The idea holds fast"
FREEDOM.
Hope! Irresistible Hope …

Oh Brilliant Triad
Person to Person
The sublime YES …

Antony Gabriel

Foreword

"Cancer is a terrible scourage, and living with and fighting cancer is a task that is truly daunting. In the rush to have surgery, radiation therapy and chemotherapy, the psychological and spiritual aspects are often forgotten. Several good studies have shown that a positive attitude can reduce stress and enhance recovery. There is also good evidence scientifically that a strong spirituality and the power of prayer can actually have a therapeutic impact on the disease.

Living with this monster, cancer, needs both a psychological and spiritual approach and this wonderful book by someone who has "been there, done that" provides a personal guide to that approach. The power of positive thinking and the power of prayer can move mountains; they can also provide healing. Father Antony Gabriel has let us go with him on his difficult journey. He has brightened this book with his wonderful sense of humour, his positive outlook, and his serenity.

I hope that his book will move all its readers to a new feeling of hope, strength and purpose."

~ J. C. Pecknold, MD

It was late evening by the time the doctor entered my hospital room for a visit I had been awaiting with a mixture of varying amounts of anticipation and dread. There would be no more speculating or Blah-Blah Bravado during which I could wax eloquent and throw around phrases showing-off my newly acquired scientific vocabulary. The moment of truth had arrived and for better or worse I would finally hear the speech. Searching the doctor's face for a reassurance not evident, I inquired somewhat glibly, "Well Doc, how long do I have?" He sat on a chair in the corner and replied with what I believed to be a practiced solemnity, "Could be two or three years; you're a C+."

Knowing that the "C+" business probably meant nothing to me, he proceeded to explain that in cancer lingo, it described a pretty serious set of circumstances. The original intruder, a malignant tumor in my colon, had introduced some bits of itself into surrounding lymph glands.

In what I assumed to be a continuing attempt to remain forthcoming, he continued his explanation that my particular type of colon cancer was unpredictable and did not always respond well to treatment. Just a few minutes before, Lynn, my wife of thirty years, had left the room. We had been waiting all day for the doctor to present the biopsy results. I needed her back to hear and later rehear of my doom through the filter of her perspective.

Lynn was back, or maybe I had only thought she was gone. Did my need manifest her presence? The doctor was explaining again but I was picking up only bits of what he was saying, " ... hit the secum ... useless organ ... spread to colon ...don't think liver involved ... hemicolectomy ... hoped we got it all cleaned out ... metastasized ... not a positive sign ... two or three years ..." My attention faded in and out, but the words, "cancer patient" remained a staple in his monologue.

Well sure, I started thinking about being a cancer patient. Of course, cancer patients have cancer, and as a priest and pastor I visited them, felt with them, comforted them and prayed for them ... pray and pray and pray.

Antony Gabriel

Someone from the church entered the room. *I don't want Lynn to drive home alone. Maybe he'll drive Lynn home, I thought. She must be upset.* What was that he said " … two or three years?" I felt I was on information overload, but that it would probably be OK. I was sure I'd be fine; on the other hand was I going to die? I was certain that all this information would be very disturbing later on when I wasn't too exhausted to panic, but right now I needed to lie here and wait for the peace that comes from being quiet.

Through all the floating I remember searching desperately for an anchor to hold me as I tried to piece together the dislocations of the past few weeks. At some point I realized it was completely dark and I was alone. Eleven o'clock ticked by, and then toward the midnight hour I picked up the phone and phoned my good friend Fr. Tom Ruffin at his home in Los Altos, California.

"Tom," I said, "guess what I just heard … " There was a long silence on the other end after my big news. Finally, he said, "I have to go." Another pause while he cleared his throat. "Let me call you back in a while," and he hung up.

I settled back somewhere outside myself to watch the emotional pendulum swing from the sense of the absurdity of it all to the sudden chill like being doused with cold water … where was my anchor? The doctor had used the statistics as he would so often throughout the period of treatment. Surgeons can be wonderful technicians but sometimes they lack the sensitivity that a patient and family so sorely need. It's the new wave. I got the facts; he left. Like Dragnet, "Just the facts, Ma'am; just doin' my job."

This is where my story begins. It is my prayer that this journal of personal struggle will give courage, hope and humor to those engaged in battle with that dreaded disease called cancer as well as any other critical dilemma. We can all identify with one another's suffering. In the understanding of our connectedness in crisis, fresh ground may be broken as we make our pilgrimage through life. Our common humanity allows us to share and bear one another's burdens.

GABRIEL'S DRAGON

I Do Not Know

I came, I know not whence
    But here I am!
I saw a road stretched out before me
    So I walked.
I will keep on walking
    Whether I wish to or not.
How did I come?
    How did I find my way?
    I do not know!

Am I something new or old
    In this world?
Am I a free soul or am I
    A prisoner in chains?
Am I leading my own life
    Or am I being led?
I wish I knew but ...
    I do not know!

And this road of mine,
    What is it?
Is it long or is it short?
    Am I going up or am I going down?
Am I the one moving along,
    Or, is the road moving?
Or are we both standing still,
    While time moves on?
I do not know.

~ Elia Abou Madey, *New York, 1938*

CHAPTER ONE

The Nightmare Begins

We had expected Christmas together to be the highlight of 1992, during which I was the pastor of St. George Antiochian Church in Montreal, Canada.[1]

The church and offices had been under renovation for close to a year, and was finally nearing completion. There would be much needed time to relax as I was close to exhaustion and pondering the future. I felt a listlessness, a general malaise in my normally buoyant spirits.

While there were many bright moments to look forward to, we were headed for the country house in Vermont with many questions concerning the past year or so to be resolved through family discussion. There seemed to be an immeasurable weight bearing down on my shoulders. The past few years of my pastorate in a large busy church had taken their toll, and my wife, Lynn, and I wanted to seek the counsel of the family about new directions. I was contemplating a career change and had begun researching a teaching career at universities in this area of North America.

Before leaving for the two-week vacation with our children, Lynn and I hosted a Christmas day luncheon for new immigrants to Canada. It turned out to be a joyful occasion with vans disgorging loads of happy passengers until mid-afternoon. Lynn had gone beyond our own community of new Lebanese to call the various consulates to obtain lists of new families living in Montreal. Christians and non-Christians alike were invited and many came. Holidays can be lonely times, especially when one is a recent arrival with no family and only meager resources. Entire families arrived in native costumes; brightly colored African attire and abundant jewelry mingled with the Arab headdresses of those crowded into the new fellowship hall at St. George.

All guests were served by parishioners of many ages. Politicians closely associated with the parish such as Senator Marcel Prud'homme joined in welcoming them. The tall, lanky French Canadian, former member of parliament, moved around the room distributing gifts. Gleeful shrieks of children receiving their gift packages of "loonies" (Canadian dollar coins) and the murmurs of their parents blended into the background of Christmas carols. The joy of all the participants warmed and brightened the atmosphere; this was never work but a labor of love. Lynn especially enjoyed planning and executing this event as a way of sharing our own good fortune and giving thanks to God for His blessings. She was like a magnet attracting donations and volunteers, and her enthusiasm was infectious, as it generated the spirit of the holiday.

As the festivities concluded we packed boxes of the remaining food for everyone to take home. The host group in the kitchen who stayed commented on how satisfying it was to share Christmas this way. Never a complaint that they had been there since the crack of dawn and still had their own family celebrations ahead of them. The youthful volunteers and drivers unanimously agreed among themselves how lucky they were to have loving homes, to live in such a prosperous country. It brought home to them that they had spent a few hours with families who had left the security of their homelands, some by choice, seeking a better future; while others had their lives disrupted by war. All cheerfully undertook whatever tasks waited to be done

The mood was warm, and as we bade farewell to the volunteer crew, we kissed them in the typical Middle Eastern fashion. This day was compensation for both the gnawing sadness within me and an unarticulated sense of frustration at the turn of events in our lives over the past two years.

Once home, everyone pitched in to help get ready for the second

Antony Gabriel

dinner of the day. Here, too, we welcomed an assortment of guests including two families who have celebrated Christmas with us since the days when our children attended Centennial Academy School together.

In addition to the traditional turkey and dressing, there were our favorite Lebanese delicacies such as stuffed grapevine leaves and baked kibbee (ground lamb with cracked wheat, pine nuts and spices). David, our eldest, sat next to me and together it seemed that we polished off the entire pot of grape leaves, cooked with lamb bones and a lemon sauce. As others had in previous months, guests commented on how I could eat so much and remain so thin. As usual my response was, "I swim every day so I burn off extra calories." In any case, my appetite was particularly hearty in keeping with the festive mood of the day.

By midnight the guests were gone, the house was quiet and it was my turn. I did my part cleaning up and packing the car with the remaining food so we could make an early morning getaway to Vermont. Filled with anticipation of the pending break I made at least a dozen or more trips up and down the many steep steps of our Outremont home to pack up the cars. I was only remotely aware of the bitter cold.

We were anxious to leave as soon as possible in the morning. Both sons were living in Montreal at the time. Mark, and David with his wife Suzanne and their daughter Caitlin, 4, were enjoying the prospect of spending time with their sister, Tammy, living in New York with her husband Bob and children Ryan, 6, and Janna, 4. Mark would be introducing his fiancé to his twin sister for the first time. Also joining us was part of our extended family, Pam Rosenberg and her fiancé.

When we arrived in Vermont on December 26, we gathered around the table for the continuation of the Christmas fare. The act of eating, especially large family meals, is not simply, for Middle Easterners, an ordinary function to dispense with as quickly as possible, but an intimate ritual of communion. It was in that spirit that we sat around the table catching up on one another's news and telling our stories.

At some point I quietly, if reluctantly, left the room. I had been running a fever and began vomiting. The consensus was that I had

GABRIEL'S DRAGON

caught some kind of severe chill while loading the cars in the below-zero weather the previous evening. My symptoms were flu-like, and my fever continued to rise throughout the night until the early morning hours. Alarmed by the fierce and incessant vomiting, which had never happened to me before, Lynn called the emergency room of the Copley Memorial Hospital in nearby Morrisville, and was told to bring me in immediately.

The family vacation, which had begun so smoothly ended like a thunderclap.

I was screaming, wracked and doubled over with searing pain in my abdomen, feeling completely disjointed. Lynn, together with son-in-law Bob and Steve (Pam's fiancé) half dragged, half carried me into the ER. By this time the pain was so intense I begged for relief. Demerol was administered and the search for the source of the pain begun. The first tests showed my hemoglobin was low, which meant a blood loss that was not evident. The attending physician advised that I be admitted for observation. The doctor on call, Dr. Joel Silverstein, was consulted.

Dr. Silverstein seemed ever present for the next five days of intensive probing to discover the reason for my symptoms. He seemed most concerned about the low blood count. I was getting large doses of intravenous pain medication and some general antibiotics in case there was an infection to fight. The immediate effect was delirium. In this disoriented state, my entire being planted firmly in mid-air, I started making telephone calls, Martha Mitchell-style, all over North America in the middle of the night. My side of the conversation went something like this, "Hi, this is Father Antony. I thought I would let you know I'm bleeding to death and no one knows why." I alerted and caused considerable alarm to many of my close associates.

I also thought it necessary to proclaim my authority to the nursing staff. "You know," I told whomever would listen, "I am a priest." I was rightfully assuming that most of them had never heard of a married priest. They needed to understand that I was very important and that they had no business trying to bring a halt to my late night phone calls. I went on to explain, "I'm a Greek Orthodox priest, but I am not Greek. I am an Arab-Christian."

— 4 —

Antony Gabriel

"Oh yeah," they'd say with a good professional Yankee-American nod, completely unimpressed by my ethnic declaration.

By December 31, Dr. Silverstein announced to Lynn that his tests weren't showing anything serious but there was definitely something very wrong as my hemoglobin was continuing to drop daily. The only exam left to be done was a colonoscopy and, though it would be difficult, he would try to assemble a team to help him get it done the next day … New Year's Day. He sought Lynn's permission to scope me, since my own responses at the time were often nonsensical. I rather liked the feeling of letting go, giving up responsibility for a while. It felt just fine not having to make any serious decisions, very fine, indeed! Thus began Lynn's role as intermediary.

I watched as the entire family came and went from the hospital room looking worried, irritatingly worried looking. I do not recall much except for the struggle to get them to understand that I needed to leave. In fact I did try to escape. I became agitated at the confinement, and despite feeling weak I pulled out whatever tubes and knobs I could yank free. I called my secretary, Nancy Calille, in Montreal to confirm my flight to a church conference in Pennsylvania the following week. I was scheduled to address candidates for Holy Orders. That was a personal commitment and an obligation that I would keep! My feverish activity meant that I had to be tackled and tied back to the bed. Failing that, I remember receiving great satisfaction from mooning my children one afternoon. "Ha," I thought to myself, "that'll teach them to imprison me."

Mark and Tammy came to say good-by as they had to return home. They were leaving with heavy hearts. The much anticipated happiness of our family vacation was over.

The professional tenacity of Dr. Joel Silverstein remained in high gear. His instincts told him something was very wrong, and, having systematically ruled one possible cause after another, he managed to find the staff on to follow through with the necessary procedure on New Year's Day. Immediately following the test he confided to Lynn that a growth was present that was somewhat difficult to detect because of its position on the Cecum at the upper end of my large bowel. He explained further that it was a solid and very "suspicious mass."

This mass, he had determined during the exam, was causing a blockage and was responsible for the pain and loss of blood. The bleeding would continue until it was removed. Surgery should take place as soon as possible. He could perform the operation or I could return to Montreal. Delicately, Lynn sought my opinion.

As soon as she mentioned the prospect of surgery, I became very aggressive with Lynn. I insisted that I had to get to the meeting in Pennsylvania. In a "me-Tarzan" frame of mind, I could do as I pleased. That included defying my wife and the doctors and nurses who were trying to convince me that I was a very sick man.

Finally, in an attempt to delay what part of me really knew was inevitable, I said I wanted to return to Montreal. Still holding to the denial, I said I would at least agree to let doctors there check to verify the situation. I did not have complete confidence in this little hospital. However, it was this hospital and its staff that saved my life.

My symptoms pointed to the flu, which I now understand is one way this type of cancer manifests. Experienced as I was at that time with the emergency room system in Montreal, especially with the shortage of personnel during a holiday weekend, I doubt that I could have received such personal and competent treatment there as I did in that wonderful hospital in Vermont. They were able to pursue the investigations diligently. I firmly believe that I might have bled to death under other circumstances before the cause of pain and blood loss could be determined.

Armed with information from Dr. Silverstein, Lynn set in motion the necessary steps for getting me to Montreal and into the hospital. She phoned my cousin Emile Shamie and told him my condition was quite serious. If I was not attended to immediately, I could die.

She wept profusely at home during her calls and throughout the night, thinking to herself that just as we had been about to embark on a new adventure, it might suddenly be over. We had gone through a great deal of late in our personal relationship, and were making plans about

Antony Gabriel

what we wanted to accomplish between ourselves, now that the children were well on their way to independence.

Over the years we had charted our course by setting short term and long term goals. This was a good part of the raison d'être for our trip to Vermont. Now, suddenly, Lynn had to marshal all her resources for a new chapter brought on by this completely unexpected turn of events.

Lynn and our son, David, who had remained with us in Vermont, brought me home from the hospital, infused with lots of medication. I was to be transported back to Montreal. That evening David and I silently watched videos. It still had not penetrated my consciousness fully. What had happened? It was as if I had been hit head-on by an out-of-control truck.

The stillness was deafening against the falling snow outside our mountain retreat. The full moon glistened and sparkled through the snow as I stared out the window, distracted infrequently by the flashing images on the television. I took refuge in our silence.

What evidence did I have of being sick, I mused to myself? In December I got lost on a familiar street in Ville St. Laurent and had to call my office to rescue me. Then I decided I was just worn out from the work I had been doing to help the thousands of Lebanese refugees fleeing the civil war destroying their country over the past five years. Then there was the building and renovation project with its attendant stress and not completed to my satisfaction. The persistent and endless conflict with the parish's lay Council over seemingly trivial issues. I had dealt with these problems by pushing down the frustration and despair I felt, and not acknowledging them, while my stamina seeped away.

My perception at that time, being ill as I now know I was, was evidently distorted. Perhaps I lacked the will to confront these issues as I had in the past, by dealing with them head-on. Oh, yes, I had also been experiencing a slight pain on my right side which I thought could be attributed to my summer's bicycling expeditions or the daily swimming routine.

Maybe a muscle was pulled. My skin had become pallid gray. Sleep often eluded me. I was eating but loosing weight. In fact, my diet was carefully planned to avoid colon disease, which runs in the family.

I managed to explain away any discomfort created by my lifestyle of working and playing hard. Being a classic workaholic-perfectionist, I simply buried the inconveniences of not feeling well to forge ahead and do the tasks that needed doing as I ministered to a large, dynamic, metropolitan parish. I paid no attention to what my body was urging me to understand.

Lynn later confided that she had noticed in the months preceding the discovery of the cancer that my life-force seemed to be slowly ebbing away. She remarked that I was like one possessed to complete each project and that I rejected all her efforts to get me to slow down. I kept telling her I was tired but fine. After all, I had just finished a battery of tests for the insurance company that indicated I was the picture of health. Nothing in the results gave any indication of what was to come.

As darkness engulfed the Elmore Mountain, and throughout that last evening in Vermont, I paced a circular path in the thick living room carpet. Feeling a desperation I'd never known, I raised clenched fists towards the darkness. Surely I was trapped in the midst of a nightmare.

Antony Gabriel

I call upon You, O God, my mercy.
You who created me, and did not
forget me when I forgot You. Let
me know You, for you are the God who knows
me; You are the power
of my soul, come into it and make
it fit for Yourself. This is my hope.

~ St. Augustine. _4th Century_

CHAPTER TWO

Surgery

It took Dr. Alan Brox, a hematologist at the Royal Victoria Hospital, no time to set up an appointment on Monday afternoon with Dr. Paul Belliveau, a renown colon and rectal surgeon in Montreal. Lynn consulted with Alan Brox by phone each evening from Vermont. He and his wife had recently received Veronique, a beautiful baby girl, from Lebanon, arranged through the St. George's adoption committee. We are childhood friends from Syracuse, New York; our grandmothers both came from Zahle, Lebanon to America on the same boat. He was instantly ready to assist us. The bond between us is so much more than professional; he is family.

Learning of my plight, a coterie of friends in Montreal wanted me transported by airplane, but I refused this offer outright. Lynn drove me, with the speedometer hovering right around 100 miles an hour, directly to Dr. Paul Belliveau's office. I do not know how we avoided the highway patrol on both sides of the border.

The nurse ushered me into the examining room. The doctor introduced himself and as I lay on the examining table, he lightly touched my abdomen which sent me rocketing ceilingward. After settling down, I asked, "Do you think I have a malignancy?" He nodded without hesitation, adding that I must be admitted immediately to the hospital. Surgery was essential, but a day or two was required to build me up in view of the blood loss and weakened state I was in.

I could not help wondering to myself, how he could be so sure, just by touching my abdomen. I was unaware that Lynn had slipped him the detailed reports from Dr. Silverstein, so this was not just a lucky guess.

When we left the doctor's office, I asked Lynn to drive me to the church office to sign a codicil to my will. Imagine the situation: I had just learned I had a serious malignancy, and my next act, even though planned beforehand, was to sign a will. Not one word was exchanged between us. Silence hung like the specter of death in the air. We were simply unable to form one intelligible sentence between us. Words that remained unsaid rumbled around in our heads. We had agreed months ago to amend the will, placing whatever assets I had under her sole custody and adding David as her co-executor.

My secretary Nancy, not knowing any details concerning my illness, had contacted us at the doctor's office to remind me that the will had been in my office for several days. I could not fathom what was going through Lynn's mind as we were riding a roller coaster which made it seem as if our lives had just been turned upside down.

I vividly recalled Lynn, during the trip to Montreal, drawing on every bit of strength in her attempt to impress upon me the deadly seriousness of my condition. I remained in my zone of disbelief, turned inward as if being closeted behind a mirror.

When I entered my office to sign the codicil, the staff had to witness the signature. I whispered to them out of Lynn's hearing that I just left Dr. Belliveau's and that my condition appeared critical. I said this as though speaking about someone else.

Once the legal business was concluded, Lynn drove me to the hospital, stopping only briefly at home to pick up a few personal effects for the hospital stay. I was admitted to the Ross Pavilion at the Royal Victoria Hospital where I spent several unsettling days prior to surgery being pumped with a variety of medicines and intravenous fluids in preparation for the surgery. Days were filled with tests, and the constant flow of visitors which irritated my family immeasurably. Their concern was for my weakened state and they wanted me to rest. They believed that people should have the courtesy to phone and ask if I could have company. For the visitors, however, I have to bear primary responsibility. The pain medication along with whatever else I was getting threw me completely off any usual patterns of behavior. I grew a particular attachment to the telephone as my link to the outside world. Looking back I see that the phone calls were a way to deny mortality and to establish that I was still very much alive and functioning as usual. The evenings as they descended brought with them the terrors of the night, terrors that remained with me for a long time.

I broke the grip of this tyranny for myself by calling friends all over North America. This was maddening to Lynn who was constantly pestered at home with such queries as, "What in the heck is going on with your husband?" Her calls to the children and our parents kept them abreast of the developments of my illness.

My penchant for the telephone elevated me to new heights of celebrity. I had already gained a certain notoriety as the "frequent caller," nudging people to fulfill their tasks. But this was different. The telephone was an umbilical cord; I was calling people to remain connected, attached and to draw strength and support.

Whenever I was free, I tried to watch television, only to be further depressed by news of Audrey Hepburn having died of colon cancer and that hockey star Mario Lemieux had just been diagnosed with cancer. I'm surrounded by cancer, I kept thinking and the next victim in line. I felt an irresistible urge to break free of this new bondage by whatever means available to me.

As expeditiously as possible, private nurses were engaged to monitor the visitors, to be available to try to deal with my whims and to try to maintain some sanity around me. Mark worked during the day so it was David's lot to maintain the vigil with Lynn at my bedside. He was studying for his doctorate in Orthopedic bio-mechanics at McGill University. With this medical background, he was keenly aware of the potential danger I remained in. A dense, angst-ridden fog enveloped my room.

Thursday morning was the appointed time of surgery. The doctors altered their schedules to attend to me as soon as possible. After I was

Antony Gabriel

informed Wednesday of the pending operation, I requested a friend of many years, Father Ihor Kutash, a Ukrainian Orthodox priest, to hear my confession and administer holy communion. He arrived around 8 p.m. Later, Father Thomas Ryan, director of the Center for Canadian Ecumenism, came by. He silently stroked my hands, as we both thought of a close friend who recently died of cancer. As I dozed off, I caught sight out of the corner of my eye, of another friend who quietly slipped in and was sitting in the corner with his head in his hands. I thought to myself, if he's in prayer, where's his kippa? (yarmulke)?

After they left, I was quite happily alone with my thoughts when suddenly a bearded priest in black flowing robes burst into my room. I asked him why he was here so late in the evening. He replied that he had only recently learned I was in the hospital and had run up to pray for me. I implored him to leave as quickly as he had come. "I have just received communion," I told him, "and need tranquility to prepare myself for what's ahead of me." He left abruptly, his hair and robes billowing behind him.

The attending nurse walked in, hands on hips and a twinkle in her eye. "Reverend, was that the black angel of death coming to fetch your soul?" I broke into gales of laughter. It had been a truly funny sight.

By eleven, I was finally alone, much to my relief, and I tried to relax. The sleeping pill kicked in and for a while I was floating. To this day I remember seeing my spiritual father, Ellis Khouri, who had died several years earlier, come into my room and hover over me, blessing me in his usual silent manner. His incandescent presence was as tangible as that of any earthling. Was this my angel? In any case, the experience left me peaceful though unable to sleep.

Before settling in, I called a parishioner who was vacationing in Florida, just to hear her soothing voice and to request prayers for the next day. We had become friends from the very start of my ministry in Montreal. Then a call to Father Thomas Ruffin around midnight. That call was so highly charged emotionally for both of us that recounting it here is too difficult to do with any amount of clarity. Suffice it to say that we discussed my condition from the now overused "worst case scenario."

I could tell he had been crying. I had been his little brother in the priesthood for over thirty years.

Throughout the dark hours that were mercifully swallowed by dawn, my thoughts flashed back over an entire lifetime, the successes and failures, the victories and the regrets. I had been a husband, father and priest for close to thirty years, and a great deal of living was packed into this time: Phoenix, Arizona; Toledo, Ohio; Chicago, Illinois; Washington, DC; and Montreal, Canada. Memory in the Middle East implies the presence of a past through an event or events, and indeed the images of the past leapt before me.

As I thrashed about in my bed, thousands of faces and events appeared, some as ghosts, some as angels, all in rapid succession until the morning light began filling the room. It came to me how much I had brutalized my own body and soul with work, struggles, conflicts, dreams and emotional dependencies throughout my ministry. I had developed a highly criticized habit of driving to the office at midnight, regardless of weather conditions, and working there alone until 2 or 3 a.m. on a daily basis.

In the ferocity of this inner turmoil, I began to have a sense of the dissonance between my public and private persona. How much of the confrontational style of my public life had spilled over into my private life? I was living on two or more levels all the time. It seems I wore my emotional buttons on my sleeve, readily available for those who knew which ones to push and when. My helter-skelter lifestyle was a continual "coincidence of opposites."

Threadlike, thoughts wove themselves in an intricate pattern within my mind's eye. Did I always do the right thing? I was drowning in a sea of self doubt. I had become a stranger to myself. Would my wife and children have loving remembrances of me or was I merely a shadowy figure who appeared out of the mist of the commitment I made early in life to the Church? Was I only a hollow functionary, a provider for the family and the network keeper for the parish? These musings are not to be confused with a "woe is me," self-centered, inward wallowing. It was a moment of truth. My head began throbbing with a myriad of images of a life that seemed to be physically and psychically short-circuited.

Antony Gabriel

I was a prisoner in a hospital bed and mired in debilitating thoughts. Tossing to and fro until dawn streamed through the window, I was longing for the anesthesia that would knock me out even for a little while. Finally, I slept for what seemed like a few minutes.

In the early morning, a team of doctors and interns appeared in the room. I felt overwhelmed in my semi-conscious state as they introduced themselves to me. "We'll do our best," they assured. They marched out as to a military beat while the orderly let himself in to shave my body, and the nurses began injecting the fluids to bring me under the subjugation of yet another power.

An ancient thinker once described hell as that restlessness where peace was unattainable. I submitted to the release of this state of being or non-being. Lynn and the children kissed me on the forehead as they were wheeling me down the hall. Their words, "We love you," floated around in my head as I struggled to hang on to them.

I mustered enough energy to tell the surgeons and nurses surrounding me in the blazing light of the operating room, "Take care of this body a lot of people depend on it; and by the way, you're going to find the first malignant tumor wrapped Lebanese-style in grape leaves!" They burst into laughter. As I dozed off, smiling, I muttered, "Bless your hands. Don't remove the wrong organ;" a strange kind of lucidity.

Half a day later, I awoke slightly in one of the recovery rooms to the soothing hands of Rose Khoury, head of nursing relations at the Royal Victoria Hospital. As a member of my congregation, Rose learned from her family that I was having surgery and volunteered to do private duty with Lynn at her side. Ice chips, wet towels and gentle strokes were angel's touches as I gradually emerged to the excruciating post-operative pain. She made sure relief was swift, kept a vigil the entire day, and was with me quite often during the two weeks I spent recovering.

Unknown to me at the time, there were a number of little dramas in which I figured centrally, taking place in the hospital corridors and a multiplicity of calls into surgery and into the church office. Speculation in the parish as to the true nature of my condition was rife. Half truths were bantered about, with reports ranging from the cancer being localized to the condition being extremely grave. These details and the distortions are still too painful to recount here.

It was some days later that I realized a major communications blow-up had occurred. While my family waited anxiously in the solarium for news from the attending surgeon, my church office was called by a member of our community who worked in another unit of the hosptial and who was somehow able to get the information by the conclusion of the surgery. He gave them an account of both the procedure and my condition. Thus my assistant knew before my family how I had fared. Lynn, David and especially his wife Suzanne were dumbfounded, and, understandably, reacted angrily to this professional breach of etiquette. To this day any mention of the incident brings a flush of anger to Suzanne's lovely face one shade redder than her hair.

I too, found this breach of privacy at such a crucial time for me, and my family, very difficult to deal with. One learns the meaning of friendship and love at such moments of crisis.

After my release from the hospital, however, it was I who received the "cold shoulder" from personnel who had resented the dressing down they received from Lynn and David, despite the fact that I was the "paralytic on the lit" at the center of this maelstrom. Later when it came time to decide about chemotherapy, this whole debacle became part of my decision to go to a different hospital.

That evening, when Dr. Belliveau visited me, he asked, "Are you the Pope or the President of the United States? Never in my surgical career has either the hospital switch board or the surgery staff had to field so many calls." I had only met Dr. Belliveau on the Monday prior to the surgery, so I was a strange phenomenon to him. "Are you so famous?" he asked. In my delirium, I responded, "Of course, yes, I am famous. Not quite the status of the Pope or the President, but famous, yes!"

"Well," he said, "I can tell you that everything went well. You did indeed have a malignancy and it took some time, but I believe we've got you all cleaned out. The right half of your bowel is gone but you have plenty left. Things look clear for now, but we'll know better when we have all the results. Until then we won't know whether or not anything else, was affected." There was more vague reassurance and up-beat

Antony Gabriel

conversation, during which we scrutinized every nuance for the information that lies in facial expression and body language. He then informed Lynn he was leaving for a surgeon's convention in California. By the time he returned the results of the biopsy would be available and the extent of the cancer would be known. So I was left hanging for a week. I descended once again to never-never land.

Through clouded eyes I was aware of the entire family hovering around me. My sister Sharon was there, too. I'm sure she could not help thinking of our uncelebrated Christmas. She had spent the holidays at their country home in St. Sauveur, Quebec until she was called to return to Montreal with the message that her brother was gravely ill.

A hard lesson: In an instant a life can be shattered forever by one of life's earthquakes. We must seize every opportunity for joy; the chance might not come around again.

When I awoke Friday morning I noticed not only the morphine pump, the intravenous and sundry other tubes invading my veins, but also a catheter. Turning to the private nurse, I ordered her to please go into the bathroom and turn on all the faucets, I wanted to listen to running water. "Why?" she asked. I curtly told her she was being paid to listen to me. She was quite understanding about my mood and did as I requested.

After about thirty minutes of listening and concentrating, I asked her to remove the catheter. Her response was, "I need doctor's orders and it is too soon. It's only one day after a major operation." I became insistent; it was my body and I wanted the thing out! She acquiesced. It felt as though my brains went out with that tube as she removed it; it was that painful. After catching my breath, the next request was that she take me to the bathroom. All the other machinery sustaining me was still attached so I was ushered in, arms outstretched, with a stiff gait, feeling as though I looked like Frankenstein's less evil twin. The nurse gently closed the doors. After a few minutes she inquired whether or not I needed help. Trembling, I implored her to come in and "… hold it for me … I want to pee."

In my mind, the faster my body began to function normally, the speedier would be the recovery process. When I completed this important task, I suggested she take me for a short walk. The medical/surgical "storm troopers" were on their way to visit me for a post-op check.

"Leave me be," I commanded as I took a few cautious, leaden steps. They looked on in what I choose to believe was amazement. For me, any movement was a miracle of independence and one that would hasten my exit from the hospital. Having had some twenty or so surgical procedures of one sort or another, I instinctively knew that I had to take control of myself. I was no stranger to a hospital environment, and my goal was to get home as fast as possible. A few mistakes in the past had taught me well. I did not want to burden the system any longer than necessary. During one hospital stay, I narrowly escaped an unwarranted second operation to remove my gall bladder. This after having had spinal surgery! Another patient with my name was in the same facility and was scheduled for that surgery. Only my vehement protests avoided this near calamity.

After any surgical invasion, the most elementary bodily function becomes an urgent preoccupation. It is the signal that the patient is on the road to recovery. I was determined not to be defeated. My body would work!

Meanwhile, despite Lynn's assiduous policing, people surreptitiously slipped into the room, causing consternation to others who, not as bold, lingered outside the closed door, and left without seeing me. A visitor's importance in some pecking order, somewhere, was perceived by its members to be related to whether or not he or she got in to see me. The "No Visitors" sign was casually disregarded. There's a difficult balance to maintain between being left alone and being overrun with well-wishers. On the other hand, families are sometimes so protective, the patient feels isolated.

I vaguely remember a friend sitting at the foot of my bed looking at me, shaking his head then looking up and asking, I supposed it was God, "Why him?" His wife had died suddenly a few years previously, and our close friendship deepened during his grief.

Two friends, a couple I had only recently introduced to each other

Antony Gabriel

after their divorces, walked in, kissed me on the forehead and left. The young woman did not at that time have the heart to tell me that she had just been diagnosed with multiple sclerosis. When I learned of this I called her from the hospital and she wept profusely, for both of us, I think.

A Lebanese diplomat appeared with his wife and son on the very day of my surgery, and was chagrined (to say the least) at not being allowed in. Lynn felt a visit from the trio, only one of whom had ever been seen by me and then only once, coming about half an hour after I got back from the recovery room was overly intrusive. "I'm sorry," she told him, "you can't go in now, he's too ill."

"Do you know who I am?" he shot back imperiously. Lynn reported her exact words as follows: "Whoever you are, he is still too ill!"

The man dropped the huge bouquet of flowers he'd been carrying, turned on his heels and departed in a huff. This kind of thing happened more than a few times. Priests dressed in black came to recite by rote the prayers as written in the book. I do not want to disparage the attempts of those good clergymen to reach me; it was just not my style. Over the years and now with even more reason, I have spoken out about the use of clichés and following the rubric when someone is lying in a hospital confronting eternity face-to-face. Often when the clergymen came to the room, they wanted to relate, to talk, and even get the update on my condition.

A person is a human being, not a condition, and it is the humanity which should be addressed by those who consider themselves spiritual healers. The formula prayers and insensitive small talk were verbal bullets piercing my head. Each time my son David sensed there was one or more (they often travel in packs) heading our way, he would rush into the room announcing, "The men in black are approaching; quick, fall asleep!"

On Saturday my brothers Philip and Charles arrived from Syracuse, as well, long-time friend Albert Joseph, who had flown in from Chicago came into the room only minutes after my brothers left. My attention span was so short and my pain was so loud I could barely accept their presence. Thankfully no one stayed long. It is an arduous struggle to attempt to be cheerful or make conversation when one's body is wracked with pain and the consciousness is experiencing a heightened state brought on by a searing new awareness of mortality.

Friends think they ought to be with you, but what they *ought* to do is ask. Solitude is the best companion much of the time.

Besides, how embarrassing it is to break wind when someone is trying to console you! That's the irony of striking a balance between companionship and feeling alone. I tried being gentlemanly when people were in my room, but deep inside, I felt my privacy was being robbed by meaningless chatter, especially in the first days after the operation. Quite honestly, I was, psychologically speaking, tied up, in knots. Beyond what was happening to me, in the moment, everything was irrelevant.

Flowers, cards and calls poured in. Senator David Angus dispatched so many flowers, in fact, that when I weakly propped my head up on a pillow, I thought I was lying in state at Urgel Bourgie Ltee, the funeral home. The calls were a paradoxical mixture of prying and genuine concern. "What's his 'condition'?" "Does he have a bag?" "Did he have a colostomy?" or "Yes, I know just what it's like," followed by a tale of the caller's own medical woes. "If you won't tell us the real truth, we have our own sources of information," was another ploy to be one of those in the know. Lynn and I had a really good laugh concerning one of the lines many callers used. When one of those came in she would run into the room and say Carol King or James Taylor (depending on whether it had been a man or a woman) just called again. In that (Taylor/King) call, at some point, the caller usually said something like this, "Listen, I really mean this, if you need a shoulder to cry on, or just someone to talk to call me any time and I'll be there for you. I mean it, don't hesitate!"

Most times, if Lynn even said so much as, "Well … " which she did once in awhile to test out the sincerity (we do bizarre things to amuse ourselves when the world starts crumbling around us), the caller would make some excuse to hang up quickly.

We used King and Taylor because both artists had great success with the song, "You've Got A Friend."

Lynn blocked my phone after surgery so she was repeatedly called to the nurses' station for incoming calls. I suddenly had a multitude of

Antony Gabriel

mothers and fathers. Family and close associates claim territorial rights when someone dear to them has been wounded and as our family unit closed in tighter around me, people who wanted information became pseudo-relatives in attempts to get the official word on my status.

Still attempting to absorb what was happening, Lynn did not want to say much. Being an extremely private person and one who is able to maintain composure in a crisis, it was not in her nature or style to speak about personal matters. At the same time it became strikingly apparent to us that colleagues and friends who feel they are close or part of an inner circle have tremendous difficulty accepting the evidence of mortality so close to them. In many, their actions showed that their coping mechanisms became somehow frozen along with any shred of sensitivity. Lynn became the one who bore the burden of fielding all the questions in addition to reassuring the family. To some parishioners, who saw her as abrupt and tense, Lynn became "the enemy." After all, I was their "Father" too!

There were, of course, the exceptions; the sensitive souls who knew how to unobtrusively convey their messages of encouragement and offer their help. They would slip quietly into the room or phone to express what good friends do, or offer sincere and kind gestures of support such as driving any family members to or from the hospital, cooking meals, running errands, (step, fetch and schlep), dropping by the hospital to keep her company or take her for a coffee and croissant break. When the offer is specific and repeatedly made, the face value is usually genuine. The others were, unfortunately, just curious, many wondering when it would be the time to hang black drapes. One must sift the wheat from the chaff. My diary is full of the conflicting impressions of these January days when my heart sank into the pit of bewilderment and despair.

Dr. Edward Tabah[2], a distant relative, came to see me on a daily basis. As a cancer surgeon, and while not my primary physician, he came as a caring friend. Other doctor-friends avoided me. I was told later that they had had access to the pathology reports, which looked grim. They were forthcoming concerning their own inability to deal with their pastor's vulnerability. Most people who knew me, either professionally or otherwise, believed I was a rock. How could someone so strong fold so unexpectedly?

Neither did the staff at the Church office, and others involved, even peripherally, with running the parish have a completely rational approach. Their responses were often entirely emotional. Senior members of the staff were shattered, and as reality sunk in, began blocking attempts of parishioners to reach me with terse replies to their inquiries, such as, "He's fine and doesn't wish to see anyone." Younger staff members were more diffident.

Those parishioners whose burdens I had borne for so long could not fathom how all of a sudden their "Father" might lay dying. Still others went into denial wanting to believe a simple explanation such as, "Oh, he probably had some simple procedure, hemorrhoids or something like that."

The national leadership of the Church I served for so many years chose comfortably to believe, against all the evidence, that I would soon be back in the work arena. Who knew better than they that Father Antony had been a fighter all his life?

In retrospect, the general disbelief and concomitant high expectations for my immediate recovery ultimately caused many daunting problems. These conflicting attitudes dragged me into a storm center, swirling around my right to privacy and my role as a parish pastor suffering from a frightening disease. In the eyes of many I was public property. At the earliest dawning of that conflicted reality, I was reminded with wonder and gratitude of having been endowed by my creator with a strong will, not only to live but to face down many seemingly overwhelming obstacles over the years.

There was no way of knowing at that time, however, that all the boundaries were being shattered.

In my semi-waking hours, I would lapse into free-flowing thought. So many memories of the past were unleashed and leapt into this semi-conscious reconciliation with my present state of being: the obliteration of the self.

Antony Gabriel

*Thou hast made us for Thyself
and our hearts are restless
till they rest in thee.*

~ St. Augustine, *4th Century*

CHAPTER THREE

Visions from the Past

Throughout my more than fifty years, I have been known as a ready combatant. As the fourth son followed by an adored sister who appeared much later; in a home filled with grandmothers, intermittent relatives boarding with us (some for months at a time and some from as far away as Brazil), an alcoholic uncle who had been interned as a POW in Guam during World War II, I had to "scrap" my way into adulthood. My older brothers were all athletes and I was the bookworm. Philip, the oldest was the artist-jazz musician; Abraham, the ardent gymnast; and Charles the artist, later to become a deputy in the Onandaga County Sheriff's department. They were all involved in basketball and football, champions at Syracuse University. Despite my place in the birth order, family economic needs and my own sense of responsibility left little time for youthful indulgences.

One of my most vivid childhood memories remains my discovery of my Uncle James, in bed, dead of an apparent suicide on his birthday. My father was devastated by his only brother's death. My mother had just given birth to my sister Sharon. Brothers Philip and Abe were away, serving in the army and the marines, respectively. Charlie was recovering from rheumatic fever and "Sito" Gabriel (my grandmother), nearly mad with grief, had given herself over to whatever release the ancient Arabic tradition of wailing could afford. I remember her shouting, a continuing litany of rhythmic pleading in her native tongue, day and night, "Where did you go, my son?" "Why did you go, my son?" "Let me go, and you stay, my son!" When she would give in to periods of intermittent exhaustion, one of her contemporaries with a son or sons took her place to keep the same mournful pace, lest the misery abate too soon, and her child be forgotten. It was a military service and Sito had to be pulled away from the coffin, still wailing. Though barely 12 years old, I remember asserting myself with an overwhelming sense of duty and propriety and the family's easy acceptance of my guidance through the funeral process as if it were the most natural thing in the world for me.

Partly to escape a household where my pre-adolescent mind perceived everyone as dedicated to invading my privacy, fawning over a new baby, worried about the boys who were away, babying Charlie because he'd been sick, still crying too much about Uncle Jimmy, and generally worried as to how to make ends meet, and partly to generate some income, I started cleaning homes for elderly neighbors. After a year or so I graduated to helping my godfather at his corner grocery store, and finally to helping run my parents' grocery store in the Irish neighborhood in Syracuse that had been dubbed "Tipperary Hill." Dad, whose English was meager, was often out at some market or other, doing errands or just in the store, delighting everyone but Mom with his good humor and willingness to share a beer or two or three, or anything else in the store, for that matter with the customers. Mom, whose idea the store was to begin with, covered the cash, and my brothers (whichever ones were home at the time) and I helped with deliveries and did what we could to make the place look like it belonged in the twentieth century. I also went to high school.

Two years at Syracuse University became the real symbol of my independence. During the summer following my second year, I took off as a kind of vagabond going from Connecticut to Pennsylvania and finally to Washington, DC, accepting invitations from different schoolmates. This was a brief two month liberation that ended abruptly when I received a call from the late Archbishop, Antony Bashir. I had been in touch with the Archbishop over the years, informing him of my intention after college graduation of one day considering attending seminary. I had eagerly received his encouraging nudges in that direction, believing that day to be some years ahead.

When the call came in early August, the Archbishop insisted that I report in September to St. Vladimir's Orthodox Theological Seminary at the Union Seminary in New York City. "Never mind university, right now," he said, "your grades are excellent and we'll put it all together for you there."

At eighteen that made me the youngest student enrolled. One of my childhood friends remarked later that I had insisted on exploding into manhood, while the rest of my friends enjoyed a more prolonged adolescence. In fact this meshed with my own constant feelings of being much older while still young.

Having felt drawn to the priestly vocation since somewhere around the tender age of five, I enjoyed the years spent rotating between Holy Trinity Episcopal Church where I served as acolyte and St. Elias Syrian Orthodox Church, my parents' home parish, where I assisted the unilingual Arabic priest at services.

To this day I do not know how or why the influence was so strong. The walls of my bedroom were decorated with all sorts of religious images and icons. The usual escapades of youth generally eluded me since my existence was so colored by the desire to be a priest. A love of the Church and Liturgical services became a defining pattern in my personal choices.

Writing in my diary compelled me to seek the person or event that sparked my interest in the priesthood. The towering figure of Metropolitan Archbishop Antony Bashir leapt from the pages to bring forward recollections of the spellbinding sermons he delivered each year during his annual summer visits to our parish. He spoke with a raspy voice using plain expressions to convey a simple message, but so charged was his persona with a divine charisma that they came to me as thunderbolts. Even a cliché like, "Where there's a will there's a way," took on a new meaning if one considered the power in the will of such a man. The diary was further evidence that it is usually a wide variety of persons, events and literary works that shape our philosophy and commitments and that we never cease to learn and grow when the heart and mind remain open to new people and experiences.

Our parents, professors and the Archbishop were shocked when Lynn and I eloped in November of 1960 in Cleveland, Ohio. Younger than myself by one year, Lynn was the first female student to break into the male bastion of an Orthodox theological school. She had somehow manipulated the system and been admitted. A striking beauty, when she walked into a room men and women alike turned to look. After two years at the seminary, we decided to get married. We drove to Canton, Ohio her hometown and later to Cleveland, where the current Archbishop, Philip Saliba, was a young priest, and asked him to marry us. At that time, Lynn's beloved maternal grandfather, Elias Esber was quite ill and not expected to live. Her mother's disappointment at not being able to give Lynn the attention and trappings of a large public ceremony at the time, had to be swallowed in obligation to her own father.

Lynn and I were best friends who just wanted to get married, no fuss, no fanfare, just be together and get on with things!

Shortly after the ceremony was completed, the priest received a call from his Archbishop wondering, "if the two crazy children" were there. He had traced our path after we left New York, fearful that a hasty marriage would eclipse our education and plans for the priesthood. He believed firmly that American-born clergy were necessary if the church was to survive in North America.

When taking the blood tests required for a marriage license, the doctor noticed something awry. Boeck-sarcoid, a tubercular disease that shows up in the blood, and about which little was known in those days was shown to be present in my test. The doctor, an older man, said that I had a rare blood disease and that we shouldn't get married since longevity was not on my side. We shrugged off his comments. We were young and impervious to anything that might stop us. In the early sixties, when we began our mission, graduating classes went forth hoping to make a difference and change the world. Idealism was high and enthusiasm for life swept us off our feet. Imbued with hope, we believed there was nothing we could not achieve.

— 27 —

Later in the fall a small tumor related to the sarcoid, was discovered at the base of my skull giving some credence in our minds to the doctor's earlier warning. Once again the choice was made to ignore his words. The tumor was removed but I was obliged by poor health to stop attending classes during my last year at seminary. In spite of the setback, I studied all through the summer to complete that final year.

During the traditional Orthodox ordination to the deaconate, the secular name of the candidate is changed to a Saint's name. I had chosen the name Elias, patron saint of my parish, but Metropolitan Antony, presiding over the ceremony changed my name to his: Antony, out of his deep affection for my family.

Following my ordination to the priesthood, we assumed a parish in Phoenix, Arizona at the ripe old ages of twenty-one and twenty-two. Naturally, the majority of the congregation was either twice or three times our ages. I have no idea why we weren't scared to death, except perhaps to say that we had heaps of yet untried faith.

A growing family compelled us to focus on providing a livable standard which in those days cost about three hundred dollars a month. The foremost goal was always to provide the best for the family and the parish. Mediocrity was never an acceptable alternative to the best. From the onset of my ministry, and often to my own detriment, I have for better or worse, been driven by my own idea of perfection.

Required by circumstances to settle in parish-owned rectories adjacent to the church in Phoenix and later in Toledo, Ohio, we lived much of our life in the spotlight. It was like being in a goldfish bowl, under the watchful eyes of hundreds of parishioners, every movement magnified for all to see. The rectory was generally considered the common property of the parishioners. We often awoke to find the "elders," several of whom possessed keys to the home in which we lived, playing cards at the kitchen table. This, we vowed, could not continue!

Following three years in Phoenix and an interim two-year assignment in Toledo, our young family moved to Chicago at the request of the recently elected Archbishop Philip Saliba. The community there had tried unsuccessfully to create a thriving mission in that major metropolitan area and the new archbishop was quick to realize this was a task I would easily and readily sink my teeth into. During this period, we became vagabonds of sorts. Being obedient to the Archbishop, I hastened to Chicago leaving my wife and three small children to live in a motel, and I had no place to call home there. After living out of suitcases for three months, our family was once again reunited. The Chicago experience remains to this day the period of the formation of many of our most intense and enduring relationships in the arenas of religion, science, medicine, the arts and, of course, politics.

We spent ten years of successful ministry in Chicago, home to the largest conglomeration of ethnic Orthodox in North America. It was there that we founded the first Pan-Orthodox Clergy Association, and one of America's first Pan-Orthodox congregations. The parish was comprised of members from every Eastern Orthodox ethnic group and many non-ethnic new converts all of whom were drawn by the common wish to celebrate the ancient Divine Liturgy in English.

Assisting us in this endeavor was the Anglican Bishop of Chicago, James Montgomery, who facilitated the acquisition of a Church building in Oak Park which was no longer used by the university community.

A parish was literally created by being willed into being. Our first services were held on a card table in a club house with twelve families in attendance. The offices of the Sheraton Center were placed at our disposal by a Montreal executive working in Chicago for a brief stint.

While in the throes of starting this new parish, I sought to satisfy my intellectual curiosity by enrolling in the Dominican House of Studies and the Lutheran School of Theology at Chicago.[3]

In the Chicago metropolitan area we developed a full range of relationships with every major political or ecumenical leader of the 1960s, the list of whom includes Mayor Richard Daly, Cardinal John Cody, Reverend Jessie Jackson, Reverend James Morton, former dean of the Cathedral of St. John the Divine in New York.

In 1970, during the uprisings in the Middle East and Black September in Jordan, thousands of Palestinians flocked to Chicago.

The small (at that time) Arab community rallied around our efforts to resettle the refugees. We were very much engaged in this effort and became quite knowledgeable about how to work effectively with the immigration bureaucracy. It was a period of immense personal satisfaction. We were needed and we were able to rise to the challenge.

Then in 1976 we were transferred to Washington, DC. Our church's presence was an active and positive force in the Chicago Community, we were in the vernacular, "smokin'!"

The Archbishop decided he wanted that same sort of image and profile for our parish in the nation's capital. He ordered us to report to that parish while he departed to the Middle East for a Synod meeting. The Board of Trustees in the Washington parish, in an attempt to assert their rights as an independent congregation, opposed our move. Some of my friends were party to sedition as they embarked on a battle with the Archbishop over the constitution of the Church as to who had the legitimate authority related to the selection and appointment of the clergy.

We'd left a lovely home in suburban River Forest on the move to Washington, thinking we'd stay in the parsonage until we found our own home. There was no accommodation for us.

Lynn and the children boarded with her parents while I stayed with my friend Tom Ruffin in the same apartment complex. We lived out of suitcases.

This unprecedented experience caught us in the crossfire as the hierarchy dueled with the parish council over who had the right to name clergymen. It was, and continues to be, an unforgettable time in our ministry, as well as a painful memory for the entire family.

After a year of politics, (why not politics? Weren't we in Washington?) the situation was beginning to look like it might be workable; the dust was settling. In spite of the fact that Lynn and I had become quite active and visible, attending many official national and international functions, we reluctantly accepted another posting to St. George in Montreal.

Lynn resumed her former job that she held in Chicago as Director of the D.C. office of St. Jude/ALSAC. This was the late Danny Thomas' pet project for cancer stricken children. The hospital is located in Memphis, Tenn. Also, we became frequent guests of the many Middle Eastern Embassies and the Ford White House. Helen

Thomas, Chief White House correspondent and William Baroody, Ford's Chief of Staff were among our mentors making inroads in the Post-Nixon era.

Long considered one of our most conservative congregations, St. George of Montreal was part of the second oldest Orthodox community in North America and one of the largest within our Archdiocese. The parish had never before been served by a liberal, socially active, ecumenically involved pastor and wife. It had also been considered for many years to be one of the foremost Orthodox communities in North America, wealthy, steeped in its ethnic roots and family traditions. It was shaped by the various village ties in Lebanon and by prominent family names. In the Montreal Orthodox community, Middle Easterners are tightly concentrated in a small area, with a high ratio of inter-marriages between clan members of the two original local parishes: St. George and St. Nichols Churches, a mere ten blocks apart. There are no secrets!

Lynn and I immediately set out to learn the landscape, the mind-set, to see what needed to be changed and what should be accepted as part of the local character. As in Chicago, we purchased our own home signaling our independence to the business people who headed the Church Commission (as the Parish Council was known in those years).

New organizations were created for the pressing needs of the community, and selected younger, or more forward-looking Parish Council members to work on administrative issues such as finances, which were in a woeful condition. Although many of the families were more than comfortable financially, the functioning of the church was taken for granted, and there was not much interest in good stewardship.

My mother-in-law Janna, gave me the nickname "Ayatollah" Gabriel on her first visit to Montreal because of all the ferment at St. George. I was doing a considerable amount of work at home. The phones at home were as busy as those in the office and I loved it! I worked at home, my mind never still. It wasn't unusual for me to accept a social invitation then spend much of the time away from my hosts scribbling notes or on the phone. This was in the days before everyone had cell phones. Janna suggested I explore the possibility of having a telephone surgically implanted to stay mobile and keep my hands free, so addicted was I to calling people late at night to check on things.

To many, the inauguration of radical reforms was refreshing. Young people were urged to take on responsibilities previously assigned to parish elders, and there was a high level of lay participation. There were signs of spiritual awakening among the young. Many felt engaged in the renewal of the church, the energy was almost palpable.

Just as the new direction was taking root and the parish expansion and building program was under way, thousands of refugees fleeing the civil war in Lebanon flocked to French-speaking Quebec. A whole new ministry shifted into high gear as the parish had to cope with the relocation of the new immigrants to Canada and all the work that such help implied; finding jobs, housing, food, clothing, medical assistance, schools, etc.

This wave of immigration was a massive assault on a community made up mostly of third generation Syrians and Lebanese, and was the largest modern-day migration to North America at one time. It required every ounce of creative energy to integrate all those who sought refuge in the church, regardless of religious affiliation.

Christians of every stripe and Muslims from Lebanon, Syria, and other parts of the Arab world came to the doors of the church seeking assistance. At one meeting alone, two hundred people showed up at the church hall after I had announced from the church pulpit that I had invited government officials to come to hear the complaints of the refugees.

Services of worship became a spectacle with so many people attending. The Canadian-born felt pushed out of their traditional seats. Some were shocked by the behavior of the newcomers. (Open breast feeding of infants during liturgy, for example, caused raised eyebrows.) In the beginning of the waves of immigration, everyone offered to help, but as the throngs swelled, so did the tensions between two very diverse cultural groups thrown together in a small space. Many of the new arrivals lacked education, because the endless war had disrupted schooling, and they arrived here without skills, without family ties, and unable to find work because of delays in processing their immigration requests.

Special emergency relief organizations were instituted to settle the refugees, and these mushroomed into a full-blown program for the parish.

Initially I had contacted the Church hierarchs in Lebanon with an offer of assistance to the young people during the worst period of fighting. Once the door was opened, the influx surpassed all expectations. More than a few of the new arrivals told me they were given three names before coming to Montreal: Father Antony, Daou Restaurant, and Adonis Grocery store. The experience of dealing with refugees in Chicago was very useful in meeting this new challenge, which far surpassed in terms of sheer numbers of newcomers, what I had tackled before.

The efforts on behalf of the refugees were consistent with my concept of the priesthood throughout the years that I had served on church committees at the national level. It came at a time when I had just signed off on responsibilities to several committees at the Archdiocesan level. For twenty-five years my work at that level, brought a great sense of accomplishment.

Admittedly, a confrontational style, boldness bordering on brashness and more than a little boastfulness did not endear me to many of my colleagues. The high profile image also worked against me. At one point I was actually told that the "brethren" resented me. Let them resent, I thought, but let them do some of the work, too. Besides, I had seized the Archbishop's vision for the church in North America as my own … I was his man!

The work in question was as Convention Coordinator, Credentials and Statistics Committee Chair, Spiritual advisor to lay groups and campus organizations. In addition much time was given to helping the hierarchy as a trusted advisor, writing, journeying to the Middle East on special missions, developing media events and lecturing at conferences and seminars.

The driving thought was always that I was the only one capable of doing the job whatever it was, the right way, so naturally, I was taken by surprise in the 1980s when I was relieved of a post which I believed I had served with considerable distinction. It was one of the responsibilities

GABRIEL'S DRAGON

I had thought about giving up because it was consuming a great deal of time and effort, but that's not the same as being relieved.

There are always signs on the trails that lead to where we are in life, too bad we don't see all of them. God speaks to us in so many languages and if we don't understand keeps trying in one way or another to reach us. The thing is we have to be still and listen or the noise and busyness keep us from hearing His voice.

Fundamental to my personal credo has always been the notion that one should never fall prey to the insipid lure of just doing the job. Two literary figures have remained inspirational in their call to action and duty, Dag Hammerskjöld and Nikos Kazantzakis. Hammerskjöld wrote, "Never measure the height of a mountain until you have reached the top. Then you'll see how low it is."

While living in Chicago I had the privilege of collaborating with the widow of Nikos Kazantzakis, Helen, on the author's posthumous work *Symposium*. During that time I was reading his book, *The Saviors of God* and took the following words from that book as my credo: "The ultimate most holy form of theory is action. Not to look on passively while the spark leaps from generation to generation, but to leap out and burn with it."

> *We fight for lost causes because we know that our defeat and dismay may be the preface to our successor's victory, and though that victory itself be temporary; we fight rather to keep something alive than in the expectation that anything will triumph.*
>
> *~ T.S. Elliot*

For the week after the operation, my mental faculties were blurred by the chemically induced stupor which had inhabited my brain. Any moment of awareness caught me in a net of self-absorbed reflection into the past.

Then Dr. Paul Belliveau's entrance into my room penetrated the interior chamber into which I had descended. Dr. Belliveau is boyish looking, with a wide grin, sparkling eyes and a charming hint of French accent in his English. "I've just returned from Los Angles," he said, "boy are you ever famous! I cannot count the doctors who approached me with inquiries about your condition. Are you Jesus Christ?" This struck me as exquisitely funny at the time.

A part of the French-Canadian milieu, Dr. Belliveau was unaware of how tightly knit is the North American Syrian-Lebanese community. It resembles, for better and worse, an extended family and rivals the rapidity of any fiber-optic cable in the transmission of bad news. Many of the doctors he spoke of were somehow connected to our community or had worked with me on one committee or another.

At all times the quintessential surgeon with a professional and ethical decorum beyond reproach, Dr. Belliveau remained discreet and gave out very little information. Since we were struggling to maintain a modicum of privacy, his sensitivity was much appreciated.

Sitting at the edge of the bed, he explained clearly and with great detail my present condition and the ramifications of the surgery from his perspective. He was blunt, as I had asked him to be, about the time frame he thought I could live within.

At that moment, I was ready with the answer. "Dr. Paul, you are not God," I said composing myself. "God does not want me yet, nor does the devil! I have spent fifty two years stirring up trouble and my job is not finished!" I was determined cancer would not disrupt my life.

The facts, however, pointed to a truly grave situation. The original tumor had metastasized and three of four lymph nodes had been affected. Once it's in the lymphatic system it's on the move and can show up anywhere.

I was still, quiet, and composed on the outside but inside everything was spastic and loud. Terror and ambivalence chased one another in my brain. At some point after I heard the word "metastasis," I could see his lips moving as he spoke to Lynn, but I could hear nothing above the mounting rumble of my own fear. Jack the Ripper stood there and pronounced my death sentence.

It had been a week since he first came to tell me that the surgery gave hard evidence to all the suspicions that I had a malignancy, yet only now was I able to realize that I had not accepted it. The instant of confirmation had arrived when all sense of security or pretenses are stripped away, when all is laid bare once and for all … no way back … I was inert.

After citing all the statistics, he said I had roughly twenty-eight days in which a decision had to be made as to whether or not I would opt for chemotherapy. He made no bones about that being the only option open to me. This meant I had to spend my time thinking about my physical self and what I wanted to do with my body. How frustrating! There were so many more important things that needed my attention! Why had my body betrayed me? I needed it to do what I needed to get done. I have no idea what it was I believed was more important at the time, I only know that I could feel control starting to give way to a sense of helplessness, and dependency and I could not let that happen!

An experimental program which was part of a research study at a medical center in Pittsburgh, PA was suggested. It was the standard protocol, my body was to be bathed on the inside with a chemical concoction of interleukin with some steroids and various other medications. What made it experimental was the addition of something called Interferon to the rest of the cocktail. Not available in Canada at the time, Interferon was said to strengthen the immune system while the chemotherapy attacked the cancer cells. The same drug was just being introduced for use in AIDS patients who had accepted to be candidates.

As other doctors would subsequently do in the coming months, Dr. Belliveau maintained that for the type of colon cancer I had, recurrence could not be ruled out by surgery alone. Although the chemotherapy would increase the chances of staying clean, the probability of a recurrence was still very much a part of my picture. Interferon, he thought, might give me some slight edge.

Lynn and I sat with tears streaming down our faces. In a staccato falsetto whine-voice I asked, without wanting an answer, "How many people have I known over the years who subjected themselves to the horrors of chemotherapy only to die having only barely, if at all, prolonged their lives? For how many emaciated post-chemotherapy patients have I prayed the granting of a peaceful release during my ministry?"

Antony Gabriel

Lynn was anxious to get me out of the hospital and on to Vermont where we hoped I could rest and regain some strength. I had lost some thirty pounds and was extremely weak from the ravages of the disease and something else.

Hardly anyone mentions or calculates the effect of what is virtually a state of death or at least a suspension of life while under anesthesia during surgery, combined with the variety of drugs poured into the body. This pharmaceutical intrusion into the eco-system that is our body surely impacts more than its target. I firmly believe, as much from observation of others as from my own experience, that this traumatic effort to purge the body, short circuits the entire nervous system.

Looking back from this distance gave me the stunning realization that a major fault line in what I had theretofore perceived as my persona, had cracked open.

I know Lord that you are all
powerful;
that you can do everything you want.
You ask how I dare question
Your wisdom
When I am without knowledge.
I talked about things I did not
understand,
about marvels too great for
me to know.
You told me to listen
while You spoke
and to try to answer
Your questions.
In the past I knew only
what others had told me,
but now I have seen You
with my own eyes.
So I am ashamed of all
I have said
and repent in dust and ashes.

~ Book of Job, *1-6*

Antony Gabriel

CHAPTER FOUR

The Questioning Begins

After two weeks, I was relieved to be released (earlier than had been anticipated) and out of the hospital atmosphere. Close friends Steve Ayoub and Andrew Auger came to fetch me and whatever accumulated loot not being left behind for the nurses and other patients. I felt quite emotional saying farewell to the nurses who had been so wonderful to me. Many had known me before the ordeal as the roving pastor who often visited patients on that floor.

Home was a welcoming bosom. Most of all I was anxious to see my ebullient four-year old granddaughter, Caitlin. Her father David had told her I was gravely ill. The interpretation in her child's mind was that I had something catching. In her preschool, she'd been taught to avoid sneezing kids. When she came to the hospital with her parents, she was very frightened by all the tubes and wires. She scuffed around my bed in her winter boots and the noise so annoyed me, I asked that she be taken to the waiting room despite the fact that I had been waiting on pins and needles to see her.

Once settled in bed at home, I called for her to come upstairs. Again she just kept walking the periphery of the room refusing to approach me. When I asked her why, she responded innocently, "Pop, you're contagious. If you die, I don't want you to take me with you, I'm too little."

I had to show her the incision and tell her, "Pop has a big cut, you can't get sick if you get near someone who's wounded."

For an instant there was a puzzled look on her face, then a smile of understanding widened between the roses that are her cheeks. She leapt onto the bed and gave me one of those wonderful squeezy hugs that a four-year old knows how best to do and planted a kiss on my cheek.

"There, Poppy, that'll make you better," she chirped as she ran out of the room.

Caitlin became the angel who would draw me back to life. I truly believe she was sent by God to rescue me from all sorts of calamities. Looking forward to and being in her presence kept me from going over the edge. My marriage with Lynn had gone through a crisis just prior to my illness. Caitlin became the link that reaffirmed our bond. In her own way she reminded us of the deep love we had for one another. Her presence was always healing, uplifting, undemanding and unconditionally loving, as it often is with little children. While she was there she only wanted to be with us, near us, by us and between us. During the evenings she spent with us she cuddled between Lynn and I as she does to this day.

"May you see your children's children … " That nurturing biblical prayer came to my lips each time I saw her. An enchanting presence releases the endorphins within us that enhance and heal.

I dissolved in an ocean of comfort in the bedroom, surrounded by my familiar icons. Lynn and the children and close friends peered in on me intermittently. Early one morning the car was packed, and, with the doctor's blessing, we were on our way to Vermont where I could avoid the deluge of well-meaning, concerned parishioners. Their pleas, "Get well fast, we need you," rang in my ears. This phrase which I heard so often in the ensuing months, did not inspire me. It made me feel I was still only a functionary and was needed only to continue to provide services. I now needed to rediscover myself.

My role as quasi-politician/priest no longer had any relevance in my struggle for life. When my closest friends emotionally asserted that it was time for me to receive and accept what I had given over the years to so many, I was overcome by gratitude and feelings of warmth. They believed life's positive rhythms would sweep away the poisonous disease

Antony Gabriel

that had eaten away at my body. They prayed for my recovery and nothing else, no mention of their own need. Knowing that felt good. I'd become stuck on the notion that I was just a functional necessity to get things done. I was like a light switch or a blender.

The fridge in Vermont was loaded with every kind of food I ever liked or even thought I *might* like. My strength and blood level needed to be rebuilt if I was to undergo chemotherapy. However, I was yet to be convinced that this was a viable solution.

Sleep evaded me at night. Daytime drowsiness was the norm. All the medications turned my daily routine upside down. Once in awhile, usually when alone in the middle of the night, I would think to myself, *I really had ... have ... cancer – **cancer!*** The very word "cancer" would dart through my head, lacerating my mind and I would catch myself wincing with the visual pain it brought.

Lynn and I watched funny videos and carried on tense conversations. We both felt uneasy about what to say, especially when the future was so uncertain. When she did go to bed, I could hear her fitful movements as I wandered through the house, convinced I had discovered a temporal purgatory.

> *Humility collects the soul into a single point by the*
>   *power of silence.*
> *A truly humble man has no desire*
> *To be known or admired by others,*
> *but wishes to plunge from himself into himself,*
> *to become nothing, as if he had never been born.*
> *When he is completely hidden to himself in himself,*
> *he is completely with God.*

> ~ Isaac of Nineveh, *7th Century*

Cancer is a dreaded word. For many it is the sound of the death knell. My father had colon cancer thirty years ago and at eighty-five was still kicking up a storm. I began to question my mother, who by now accepted quite stoically, as elders tend to do, that I had a cancer operation. She was quite clear on the fact that Dad had no chemotherapy. His cancer was surgically removed, but this established that colon cancer was most likely familial.

Many of my clergy friends wanted to visit, but I insisted this would be impossible, Vermont was to remain as a place of refuge and quiet, not a center for entertaining which was sure to be the case if some of my brethren made the trip. Lynn was too preoccupied with me to have to cope with an expanded household. In addition I could barely tolerate the presence of anyone, except Lynn, in the same room. My noise irritation antenna was at its zenith. Some Montreal and New York friends made day trips and while it was pleasant to see them, talking and laughter seemed so harsh a penetration to my ears, I was often driven to distraction. Needing solitude to sort out the rapidly changing events, I frequently retreated to the bedroom if there were visitors; body and spirit still quite fragile.

Few past the age of forty can claim a complete history of perfect health and I most certainly had not been one of the few. The presence of the Boeck-Sarcoid disease, noted at the time of our marriage, has always meant my immune system was compromised. In 1989 it left me wide-open to the ravages of a wild prostate infection that ended in my being laid up for weeks with extreme toxemia. There were other times when what I thought might be a simple ailment seemed to get out of hand. I had always managed to land on my feet. Not ready to accept any explanation that didn't confirm my invulnerability, I became irritated with the fact that physicians, invariably, pointed to stress and overwork as the cause of a vulnerable immune system. A good cop-out, I thought! Pretty nervy to always blame the guy who's sick for being sick.

The days were eating one another, and I gradually regained more strength. The cold weather of January and February almost precluded any outdoor excursions. Lynn, however, occasionally bundled me up to drive the scenic mountain roads. The glistening white snow against the splendid blue sky was a breathtaking sight. Had it been here last year? The fresh, crisp air seemed of its own volition to be breathing into me the very *essence* of life, could the elements do that?

Back at the house the familiar preoccupations of "Why me?", "Why

Antony Gabriel

now, and how?" would be waiting for me, jealous of the hour I'd enjoyed without them. The belief persisted that if I focused on the causes I could find some answers and that might somehow put the demon disease under control. It could have been familial, in the genes, a predisposition, like my father; it might have just happened like an explosion in my body; maybe the Boeck-Sarcoid had something to do with it; possibly a stressful lifestyle was at fault; more likely my colon was just weak; then, again ….

None of this served any purpose except distraction from having to make a decision about chemotherapy. My initial reaction was negative, but my whole decision-making process was immobilized; alienated from the resources from which I normally drew strength. The wellspring that had enabled me to reach out to so many people in some kind of physical or emotional pain seemed to have run dry.

———————————

But love whose cause is God
is like a spring welling up
from the depths: its flow never abates,
for God alone is that spring of love
whose supply never fails.

~ St. Isaac The Syrian, 7th Century

CHAPTER FIVE

Reflections on a Priestly Life

As I had begun doing in the hospital, I spent the next several weeks in Vermont rummaging through the compartments of my mind, checking for clues. It seemed vital to find any map that my conscious or subconscious mind might have squirreled away that would lead me to this discovery. Bearing in mind that one can be only so objective when viewing one's self through one's eyes, I thought I was looking at some pretty great stuff!

A charmed life, for the most part, however tumultuous, it was still a charmed life, reviewed and censored by my ego's strict blue pencil. I saw it as follows:

> Finished school early, ordained at a young age, married a creative woman with her own career. Had great kids who gave us little trouble; fortunate, considering the turbulent times.

I was an overly confident high achiever; recognized no limits and set few boundaries even in engaging myself with others. I was pretty sure that I had the solution to everyone's problems; they needed only to ask, my grab bag was full and ready. I assumed or appropriated everyone's hurt or pain as my own. This resulted in many rough spots along the way, but God had gifted me with tenacity, therefore, I would surmount any challenge or attack – eventually.

Always believing myself a cut above the rest, I was, in brief, bold and brash. I have also been known to be obnoxious, enjoying the accolades heaped on me and proud to be considered, "The man who gets things done." My sincere belief that I was the best at whatever I did was difficult to hide since behavior and attitude always belie any pretense of humility. How could one be humble and at the same time be *the* priest who inaugurated unique and revolutionary situations through the Church? Furthermore I could not ignore the fact that I had achieved some measure of success in the secular world as well. I was now in my fifth year as professor at McGill University's Department of Religious Studies where my course "Eastern Mysticism in Contemporary Literature" was always filled to overflowing.

I was, after all an urban priest, and it requires special skills and more than a little dynamism to maintain the multi-dimensional aspects of each parish, especially in the context of the many shifting values that were unsettling society. Being told constantly that one is a charismatic leader ultimately leads to higher inner expectations. It is possible to forget that one's feet *do* touch the ground. Nevertheless, a priest is entrusted with the spiritual lives under his charge and there are no real pinnacles of the profession in the ministry of healing as in the secular world.

Although she became in more recent years a fierce, at times, ferocious, guardian of our personal lives, Lynn has always been there pushing me to the maximum. She was the dreamer in the family; I merely put the framework to many of her visions. The original manuscript of this work included a portion on Lynn's background and spoke much of her work and accomplishments. There was even an anecdote or two from our earlier years. With respect to her wishes that portion has been omitted. Suffice it to say, that if ever I soared above the mountains, it was on Lynn's blithe spirit.

In all the parishes where we ministered, my work patterns have been the same, feverish, relentless, and something akin to a clerical octopus with tentacles. I brought with me to Quebec my habit, formed in the earliest days of ministry, of visiting the homes of every known

Antony Gabriel

Antiochian Orthodox family. Whether somehow attached to my parish or unchurched, if they lived in the Province, I found them.

No matter how exhausted I was, how awful the weather conditions, how many times I got lost, I *visited*! Sometimes a parishioner or two who knew the area would accompany me, but more often I was alone. Visiting as many as twenty homes in a day, I crisscrossed the city lest I miss some nook or cranny where a member of the congregation or someone who might need me, might be.

After many years of following the same routine, a recurring pattern emerged which seemed to point to a real dichotomy in my ministry. Far too often there was little, if any connection between my visitations to parishioners and their participation in the liturgical life of the church. While I was always received with hospitality and courtesy, at times even lavishly so, there was a gnawing sense of dissatisfaction when the hospitality and courtesy did not translate into responsible involvement in church activities.

Ignoring the uneasiness, refusing to believe that my formula could be flawed. I continued with my *mission*. At times even while visiting, I felt my priesthood somehow diminished to a position more like one of guru/courier for the Spirituality Home Delivery Company. Still I persisted with the home visitations like some sort of pastoral sorcerer's apprentice.

It is typically Canadian to be ritually and traditionally drawn to the church for the rites of passage, but unlike the American situation, there is little widespread sentiment for regular weekly attendance. As a result I instituted all sorts of commemorative Sundays to draw people into the church. Monthly memorials, marriage rededication ceremonies, lay sermons, recognition for many organizations with their liturgical participation. The Church even boasted three choirs; one for Byzantine music, another for the youth and a large English choir, as well.

Just prior to my illness, I began to sense the strain of so much *doing*. In midnight dialogues with myself, I kept mulling over and over possible reasons for my new feelings of vulnerability. One Sunday afternoon only a week before Christmas, I went to visit a severely ill parishioner at the Montreal Neurological Institute. After the prayers, I lingered in the corridors with the man's sons-in-law. The conversation turned to the state of affairs in the parish. In an unusual turn of events, as much a surprise to me as to my sympathetic listeners, I found myself seeking their intervention in what I perceived to be personal attacks in the parish. I told them I thought there was an orchestrated campaign by some in the parish to undermine my authority. This was the first hint that the information from my internal dialogues were becoming too loud to ignore.

During the previous year a new Parish Council had assumed responsibility over the business of the parish, and several of the members were from families with whom we had formed personal relationships. Over the many years a genuine team spirit had developed based on a sense of mutual trust and a continuous give and take of ideas. Disagreements were settled in-house and with considerable respect for one another's opinions. My familiarity with the new Council members contributed toward my being lulled into a false sense of security. When a faction of the congregation began to stir the rumblings that the priest was too domineering, that he tended to control everything, and that the new Council would be rubber stamps for the approval of the priest's wishes, I was quick to dismiss such grumbling as the nonsense it was. That task was much more difficult for those whose actions and opinions were challenged because of a relationship to me.

At that time the issues on the Council's table included acquiring a competent staff, building and renovation, and programs responding to the various religious, social and educational needs of the parish. In addition there was still the huge wave of immigration because of the continued fighting in the Middle East. Believing that agenda enough for any working group, and given the harmonious track-record of its inner workings there was no reason to consider anything that did not broaden our image and outreach. Unaware that the new Council members were constantly torn between a loyalty to the projects that had been initiated and the pressure to demonstrate an independent will, I continued to pile on responsibilities.

Antony Gabriel

At my insistence, an interdenominational body composed of area Christian and Moslem leaders was created. This became a viable organ that created an immigration fast track for people languishing in various countries. Thousands of dollars from the parish budget were allocated for emergency aid. The Helping Hand Committee was formed under the auspices of the Antiochian Women's Organization to help meet the seemingly endless demands on parish resources. Later, the Societe de Bienfaisance de l'Eglise St. George was set up, and under it the Adoption Committee worked to clear the way to bring children to Canada for adoption.

We pestered the media and the Ministers of Immigration to alleviate the untold personal suffering of the Lebanese. I dealt with all levels of government to help reunite families, stop deportations, release political prisoners from incarceration, using every political association to serve the community's needs.

One day an official from Ottawa called and said, "Okay, Father Antony, 500 sponsorships to Canada from Lebanon, Greece and the United States are quite sufficient! How many people are *really* working at your church?"

The 500 family mixture of mostly Canadian or Egyptian-born congregants burgeoned to nearly 2000 families with the addition of the throngs of immigrants from throughout the Middle East. We were hosting multiple services, and there were more organizations than ever knitting the new Canadians together until the time would come for them to inaugurate a new, separate mission. It was the general feeling that the day would eventually arrive when this body would be a self-sustaining spin-off with the blessings of its welcoming hosts.

In my own single mindedness of purpose(s), I lost sight of the fact that no matter how noble, no single-minded vision is ever accomplished single-handedly.

Sheer force of my will was not equal to the task of uniting the private agendas of new immigrants wanting their own place and voice in the community, and, the descendants of the founding families who thought everyone should be in full support of the huge renovation project under way. Both groups were disappointed in the feeling that I had deserted them to give more attention to the cause of the other. At the same time I knew I was more fully involved in both causes than either faction, having been the initiating energy behind both goals.

Those I had moved heaven and earth to help, folded their tents and stole away in the night as I slept. Some of the new dissenting immigrants were incited to leave St. George and establish an Arabic speaking parish on their own before telling me. Didn't they know I would have helped them at the proper time?

My *friends* on the Parish Council showed me they were in charge. The renovation project was completed and a celebratory banquet was held replete with effusive congratulatory speeches by the Council members for *one another*. I do not recall one word of acknowledgment of my part in initiating the project, obtaining the property, or channeling government funding and private bequests to the church. My vision had been appropriated as their own and I was ingloriously ignored, asked to present gifts of gratitude as the committee took their bows. Or, this is how it seemed to me at that time, or was it my perception?

These were crushing blows to my psyche, the fragility of which was stretched beyond anything I could ever have suspected. I stubbornly ignored any sign that even my own body was conspiring against me by incubating destruction in my very bowels.

That many of my activities seemed to be under critical review effected no change in my behavior. It was no one else's business if I had undertaken to organize and supervise the funding of a choral society outside the parish to benefit a young man whose talent seemed to me to be extraordinary. Neither was it reasonable of parishioners and family to believe that my agreement to host a weekly radio talk show was, in addition to everything else, way too much. Something was very wrong! Something inside me was not being fed fully or quickly enough. I needed more and more recognition to bolster my flagging self-esteem and when I got it, I needed still *more*. My flock and my loved ones felt deserted and replaced by my pursuit of outside interests and adulation. How narrow of everyone! How plebeian not to understand that these things gave a broader dimension to my ministry.

Antony Gabriel

How easy it is to recognize from the distance of a few years that normal reasoning processes and underlying rational behavior were suspended somewhere outside and beyond my perview. Instead, my fantasies of control and self-aggrandizement preserved a powerful illusion about who I was and what was expected of me.

I had found the crumpled, discarded map hidden away in a corner of my sub-conscious. If the old saying, "There are no secrets in the unconscious," is true, and I now believe it is, there was surely part of me that knew I was in big trouble. The information was there, I had simply made a choice to read it differently. The message I'd been given was:

"If you are here you need help. Stop. Look around. You are flesh, you are weak, you are ill, you are lost. This is the road to Ignominy and Destruction. God has the direction you need. Please seek His guidance before continuing." But the way I read, was, *"You have reached a difficult place, but you are steel. You are strong. You are invulnerable and wise. You are a tireless giver of your gifts and talents yet your work and genius are not appreciated. You deserve love and recognition as did Jesus Christ. Your journey has been much the same as His. Ignore all but your own counsel. This is the road to Vindication and Validation."*

All the while the melodrama of my life was playing inside my head, the tumor was nesting in my body and the parish routine with its real life joys and tragedies continued. Marriages, baptisms, illness, death and divorce claimed my energies.

Conflicting expectations of my role, or, for that matter the role of any pastor tumbled together in my head. I replayed the following attributes of a clergyman as viewed by his determined detractors:

- A strong voice; too boisterous
- A soft voice; too timid
- Drives a nice car; too materialistic

- Drives a modest car; doesn't represent community well
- Has a strong will; too egotistical
- Shows humility; too wimpy
- Has a sense of humor; too silly
- Insists on seriousness; too dour
- Dresses well; too sophisticated
- Doesn't dress well; too disheveled
- Calls a parishioner; what for?
- Doesn't call; doesn't care
- Loves the elderly; neglects the youth
- Spends time with youth; neglects the elderly
- Prays obviously; too pious
- Not seen in prayer; too secular
- Active wife; she's too bossy
- Wife not active; doesn't help her husband
- Appears hearty; not working very hard
- Appears not well; check out replacement

A stark, most unwelcome revelation forced itself on me in the restlessness of the moment. I had failed myself and my congregation! I was exhausted and had become mute in the face of adversity. As Octavo Paz so succinctly observed, "Glory is a frequently miscalculated goal and oblivion can get the better of any reputation."

Antony Gabriel

I will extol You, O Lord. For You
have lifted me up.
O Lord, my God, I cried out to You
and you healed me.
O Lord You brought my soul
up from the grave;
You have kept me alive,
that I should not go down to the pit.
Weeping may re-enter for a night
but Joy comes in the morning.
You have turned for me my
mourning into dancing:
Thanks to You forever.

~ Psalms 30

CHAPTER SIX

The Decision

*T*he din of my thoughts subsided at some point that evening. I do not remember whether it was a gradual tapering of the carping litany of my inner critic or a swift rescue from its harangue by the merciful intrusion of sudden stillness. However it came about, I knew its Source and was suffused with gratitude as I noticed myself gazing at the winter sky.

The wall of glass doors leading to the gallery offered so perfect a view of the stars on their endless navy blue background, that I felt no separation from them. There were so many, they were so bright so near, all around me. I was among them. "We are part of the stars" was the thought I took with me as I drifted into a dream. The watcher in me observed myself as a traveler sailing past hundreds of the twinkling lights of various sizes. There was a look of grave determination on the traveler's face. He had somewhere very important to go. The watcher wanted the traveler to slow down a little to prolong the sense of exhilaration that always comes with one of those dreams in which we can float or fly. At the very instant I had wished it, he slowed. I hadn't said anything. He was ready and willing to comply with my unspoken thoughts with no hint of reluctance or hesitation. Still, as the watcher, I knew that slowing the pace had been a huge concession on his part. Then looking over at where I was (or where I would be if I had actually been there), the traveler flashed the watcher a heart-melting smile. The smile was totally indulgent without being condescending and something in it let me know that he had a special destination in mind. The destination would be more wonderful than I could imagine and it promised to be a delight for all of my senses. I trusted him completely, although I had no idea what he meant, and I made a conscious choice (as conscious as any choice can be while one is asleep) to enjoy the ride.

We moved swiftly and purposefully, yet completely without a sense of urgency. From time to time a star or two would swerve to avoid us as we journeyed. How *confident* was this guide. How absolutely I trusted him! I remember thinking ... *this is like falling in love!* At that same moment I felt wracked with laughter at the silliness of falling in love with myself. *I* was not laughing, I *felt* laughter and I began to sense our destination was near. At that moment a tiny thrill sought entry to my being and at the instant I thought to bid it welcome, I drew in a breath and bliss was everywhere. I *was* bliss. For a while, a length of time I have no way of measuring, the stars kept reconfiguring themselves in rapid kaleidoscopic shifts until they finally formed themselves into a path. As I took the first step on that path, my only thought was, *I am safe; I want this feeling to last forever!*

The star-path lead to the Convent of the Presentation of Our Lady in Beirut and to the two nuns there who are my distant cousins. In reality that convent had provided a safe haven during a long-ago trip to Lebanon when several failed attempts on the lives of our group had been made in hopes of thwarting a mission we were there to accomplish.

I followed the path to the chapel where I saw myself on my knees as Mother Mary-Jo and Sister Belagia chanted prayers for my health. I continued watching, enraptured, as they each gave me a piece of blessed bread dipped in rosewater. So famished was I for some tangible sign of hope that I eagerly opened my mouth to accept the offering and as I did so I actually tasted the honeyed bread. As I swallowed I both saw myself and felt bathed in the sweetness of their act, the steadfastness of their faith, and was swept away by the haunting beauty of their voices repeating the ancient chants. It was a fleeting moment of exquisite tenderness, the memory of which abides with me to this day.

— 55 —

When I awoke, I related the dream to Lynn and asked whether she thought it might be some sort of sign. At that time, I was the only one with any question in mind as to whether or not to opt for chemotherapy.

Lynn leapt at the opportunity to influence my thinking in that direction, "Of course it's a sign! How much clearer could it be?" I knew, however, that Lynn was already convinced and so anxious for me to agree, she would have sworn that dishes in the sink were a sign.

The next day I received a phone call from a friend in Paris, Nabil Nahas, on his way back to Montreal from Lebanon. He had a gift for me from my cousins, a loaf of holy bread! Mother Mary-Jo and Sister Belagia had reached across six thousand miles in a dream to revive my spirits, using the homey, simple symbol of bread, so basic in the cultural language of Middle-Easterners.

My vacillation ended and Lynn was much heartened by the decision to proceed. She phoned Dr. Belliveau in Montreal and asked him to make the necessary arrangements. He expressed sincere relief at our decision and urged us to return immediately.

In the announcement to Dr. Belliveau that we were prepared to be initiated into the new rites of sacrifice for life, there was one condition, a change of venue. While at the Royal Victoria Hospital, I had had only sporadic periods of rest because of the continuous traffic through my room. The sprawling old Royal Vic, or just the "Vic," as it is affectionately referred to by most Montrealers, is the health care institution most used by our community in the city. The hoards of visitors, no matter how well-meaning, often became intrusive. In addition, my stay had become political. Small victories were recorded by those who gained entrance to my room; and losses by those who did not.

We decided that I would go to the Oncology unit at St. Mary's Hospital. For one thing, I was somewhat less well known there, and secondly, a factor which later proved to be a blessing, as a Catholic hospital it provided a religious ambiance. Another consideration which doesn't even enter the process when a life and death decision is being made but has real, practical value once one is slogging along through the winter slush, was parking. The security man turned out to be most compassionate and we went door to door without charge, keeping warm and dry.

Antony Gabriel

Dr. Belliveau informed us that he was associated with both institutions as a part of the McGill teaching hospital community, and he contacted Dr. Peter Gruner, Chief of Oncology to make the necessary preparations and transfer my file. Evidently I had arrived in the nick of time. The deadline was soon to pass for admission to this experimental protocol. A few days later we were called to come in on Friday for a consultation with Dr. Gruner at the regular weekly meeting of his team. I had been accepted as a candidate. I wasn't sure, however, that it called for rejoicing since it wasn't exactly like graduating to something or from something.

Then another hurdle popped up. How to find a new vein every day to pump the medication into me? Fortunately, a cousin, Karen Habib, a nurse, called from Florida. When she learned about my forthcoming treatment, she told Lynn that I should insist on a porto-cath to give a continuous direct line into my bloodstream for the chemotherapy. This would skirt the necessity of having to poke a new hole every time. A phone call was made to the surgeon who performs the procedure, the request was made and I was scheduled to have the permanent access made on the same morning the chemotherapy was to begin.

The medical team explained to Lynn some facts (as it turned out, the information given was incomplete and far too scant) concerning the protocol I would be receiving along with explicit instructions as to how to administer the Interferon injections. My routine was to be one week on chemotherapy and three weeks off for six consecutive months. During chemo week, Lynn would give me the two Interferon shots on weekends; the rest of the time I would receive the shots at the hospital before the rest of the protocol was started. Next she signed the consent papers agreeing, as well, that we would be responsible for payment, since this protocol was yet to be accepted by the Quebec Medicare program.

I just listened to it all like some sort of slinky-toy with ears, poised at the top of a great stairway, about to embark on an end-over-end, non-stop, downward journey that would take me on a swift trip to a place I'd never been, didn't know if I wanted to go, and wasn't sure I would make it back. Even if I did get back, how much of the man who did survive would still be me?

"Please, God," I remember thinking, "could You just take charge for awhile? I'm tired, and I don't feel very well, and I do not know what's going on!" I suppose it was actually a prayer, but at the time, it felt more like asking a really good friend to do me a favor because I was temporarily in a spot and I was sure that friend would understand and help. Now that I think about it, that's *exactly* what a prayer is! (Or at least one of the things a prayer is meant to be.)

> *Faith is the gateway to mysteries.*
> *What the eyes of the body are*
> *to sensory objects the same is*
> *faith to the eyes of the mind*
> *as they gaze on hidden treasures.*

~ St. Isaac, *The Syrian, 7th Century*

I crawled into bed immediately after returning home from the Friday meeting and stared at the ceiling until early Saturday morning when Lynn appeared with my first Interferon injection. Initially she was timid with the needle, but the pharmacist had given her extra needles so she could give me a double dose for the first time. Once she mastered her energy and nerves, she plunged that dreaded needle straight into my hip and it was she who said, "Ouch!" as she would with every injection for the next six months.

Almost as quickly as the needle was retracted, I began reacting as if I had a bad flu bug; shaking all over and feverish. A call was made to the Oncology Department to ask what should be done. The reaction was to be expected, they said and recommended Tylenol. Why hadn't someone said something before about what could be expected, and what might be recommended? So chills, fever, aching joints and Tylenol were the first part of the drill I would become so familiar with. That Saturday and Sunday, however, I spent sweating in bed, picturing the coiled slinky that connected my head to my feet, bobbing down a bottomless staircase.

On a frosty February Monday morning at 6 a.m. we left for the hospital accompanied by Magid Tarabulsi and my sister Sharon. I was

Antony Gabriel

dressed in a cap and jeans feeling like a candidate for some labor camp.

Magid Tarabulsi was one of the graces of my illness. He materialized out of the network of parishioner friends and offered with amazingly firm, yet gentle insistence to accompany me to chemotherapy. His support was constant and steadfast and never overbearing throughout the entire six months. He chose the exact moments when he was needed to appear and never lingered without reason. A larger-than-life elf whose presence brought care-filled concern and a fleeting sense of order to a chaotic period in my existence.

The pipeline to my bloodstream was surgically implanted in my chest and I was rolled into oncology where chemical cocktails of all sorts were being served. I glanced around the room and saw several beds now filled with more patients. We, "the slinky-toy people," were introduced to one another. This section of the hospital was to become my temporary home and the chemo-companions a new kind of family. Oh well, I supposed I could handle it easily enough. However, as soon as the drum-like top of the pipeline was punctured and I looked up and saw the clear fluid begin to drip slowly into me, tears rolled onto my cheeks. The feeling was not so much crying as that of emotion leaking onto my face as the liquid poured in through my chest.

Who did Alexander Solzhenitsyn and Boris Pasternak think they were with their Gulags and Cancer Wards and Zhivagos? No! That wasn't the question I wanted to ask! Why had I the temerity to believe that merely having read these works admitted me to the ranks of the cognoscenti? Reading the descriptions of horror and misery, allowed me to believe I felt the fragility of Everyman, that I had been intellectually and spiritually enlightened as I admired the prose and syntax of the authors.

Living my own Gulag and Cancer Ward, I watched the scales fall from my eyes and saw that language is only a rudimentary tool in the human effort to communicate and that even in the hands of those who know best how to use it, it is a puny thing compared to any need it seeks to convey.

Lynn and her cousin, Jeannie Habib, were at my side wanting to hold my hands, to give me something to sip or to try soothing me into stillness as my limbs trembled in mockery of any notion of control I might still harbor. Melancholy overtook me and I continued to leak my silent tears.

At that moment I began to learn the lesson that my body and its will were waiting for me to claim the wholeness that would help create my own healing and would teach me much about my relationship to God. If I could not command the functioning of my flesh, I would try to fathom its mysteries!

Having spent the requisite time wallowing in as much misery and discomfort as my limits would bear, I determined to do what I could to introduce whatever pleasantness I could to whichever of my senses would accept it. My first thought was of sacred music. I would get a small tape player with a headset and pass the time listening to sacred music. One day a friend called and asked whether I needed anything and without hesitation I said I needed a walkman.

The word went out and tapes of Byzantine chants, choral works, and the masses of Faure, Bach, Mozart, and Beethooven were delivered. Someone sent Arabic chants by Sister Marie Kayrouz of Lebanon. Her voice was clear and poignant against the background of the oude, a Middle Eastern guitar-like instrument, and the flute.

My new resolve to pay closer attention to the messages of my body was already creating dividends. My spirits mellowed to the rhythm of the chants and orchestrations and in this manner, the long tedious hours in the oncology unit passed a little more quickly. It occurred to me as I continued to listen to the tapes at home that this was a marvelous way to harmonize the body and the spirit. As the months passed, I recommended this practice to others whom I believed needed help in coping with the ordeal of healing under the assault of chemicals.

If one visualizes the power of music as it flows in synchronization with the healing powers within, it can become a source of restoration and renewal. Even while sleeping, music seeps into the soul and neutralizes agitation. Beauty saves, I thought so often to myself, therefore, we must glimpse as much as possible in nature and open our souls to its vibrations in music.

Antony Gabriel

As one learning and finding myself in circumstances so foreign, I could easily have been in some parallel universe. I discovered new truths at every turn and often in a most unlikely medium. Old adages or axioms even what seemed tired clichés, often seemed like newly discovered truths. I learned that there are no guarantees and nothing is for certain. At the same time I knew one thing for sure. Every effort can be creatively exerted or converted to combat depression and the disease which is its source. Music is a therapeutic tonic to still or soothe the heart and mind and subsequently elevate the spirit. Although each day was a new struggle to continue, I decided to create a new reality.

After the first chemotherapy session ended, Lynn and I were taken to Florida by close friends Larry and Cookie Rossy. I rested in their lovely condo in Fort Lauderdale for a week or so during which many of our acquaintances who spend the winter months there were quick to call with invitations for lunches and dinners. Even though many of the invitations were from people with whom I never had much occasion to socialize with, I wanted to accept them all. Lynn and our hosts just assumed that my judgment was somehow impaired and simply put a lid on things by saying, "No thanks," on my behalf.

I resented being handled and yet, at the same time was grateful that someone put the brakes on for me. I was always willing to push myself, but I was honestly tired. Never willing to admit to the reality that every outing exhausted me, I just didn't have any reserve energy.

One good day we walked the beach. I had been told to avoid the sun during the months of chemotherapy, and took some rather childishly perverse satisfaction in walking under the blazing Florida sun. I remembered having promised myself that I would create a new reality, but I'd get to that later. That particular day, in a spontaneous affirmation of life, we all swam, fully clothed, in the ocean. Swimming was invigorating and reassuring. That Lynn and our dear friends had joined me provided a sense of secure connectedness that was only fleetingly available to me these days, or so I thought.

Later several of my doctors conceded that they believed my swimming over the years contributed to the rapid pace of my recovery, since exercise helps to stimulate and strengthen the immune system. I had been an obsessive swimmer for over ten years, at least five days a week, no matter where I was.

During the several "off" weeks in Vermont, a friend arranged for me to use the spa and pool at the Topnotch Resort Hotel in Stowe. There I would swim, receive massages and relax in the hot tubs, all healing activities in the new reality I was constantly recreating for myself. Often, nearly hypnotized by the shafts of winter sunlight coming through the skylight and sparkling in the indoor pool, I felt bathed in the reflected glow as I submerged myself in the warm water as in prayer.

I found swimming to be a spiritual experience. Underwater, I understood clearly the Byzantine theologian Symeon's colorful description of the mystical encounter. The simile he used was that of a diver who plunged into the depths of the Mediterranean, and was so absorbed by divinity that the shore disappeared. As well, in the rhythm of the strokes, one can meditate or pray without distraction and therefore coordinate the heart and breathing with the Divine Name. The symbol of water in religious parlance is that of renewal, a powerful life force.

> When a man walks into the sea up to his knees or waist, he can see the water all around him. But when he dives into the water, he can no longer see anything outside, and he knows only that his whole body is in the water. This is what happens to those who plunge into the vision of God.
>
> ~ Symeon, 11th Century, *The New Theologian*

Antony Gabriel

CHAPTER SEVEN

The Descent

It would be impossible to adequately describe or chronicle what transpired during the next five months of treatment. The period from March through the end of July passed sometimes at a snail's pace or raced ahead as if on fast forward depending on which reality I was creating at the given moment. I realize with amazement how one can disassociate the self from pain or discomfort. It is also one of the many great blessings we are given that the mechanisms of memory depend entirely on choices we make, whether consciously or by default. This explains how a mother forgets the agony of childbirth as soon as she sees her baby. On the other hand, when in the middle of a bog of despair, one can experience a slow sinking and weakening as one is slowly pulled down by inexorable forces. Thus we spent six months alternating between the hospital and our residence and country home; alternating between hope and despair.

The Chemo week became a ritual in which survival became my entire preoccupation. When I returned home from the early morning to mid-afternoon chemical infusion, after walking and resting, I became restless and sought to include parishioners and friends in early evening soirees. I felt compelled to call and urge anyone who had wanted to visit me, but had not been able to while I was in the hospital or in Vermont, to visit me now, in my home. Busy businessmen would leave their affairs to rush over when I returned home; women from the community came by, food in hand, for afternoon tea. I felt their genuine concern for me and my prospects for recovery. I regaled them with funny hospital experiences or stories from my priestly ministry. My need for an audience was tantamount to my desire to make a statement that I was still here, that my whole self had survived, would continue to survive intact. By laughing at my own foibles, in the company of visiting parishioners, I was still functioning in the role of teacher with the lesson that it was okay to be human. This was also a way of putting unpleasant experiences into perspective, and sometimes to help turn them around.

All of this contributed to Lynn's anxiety about my energy being sapped while I was performing, no matter how much she liked the families that came by. Sometimes friends called to take my father-in-law and me out for supper, especially if Lynn was in Vermont.

My father-in-law, Nick Georges, had come in answer to Lynn's plea for help in managing me. Nickie was a no-nonsense straight talking man who had had two malignant tumors removed over the past ten years. He never looked back and never complained. We had always had a great relationship and his rapid-fire sense of humor, no matter the situation, made his company a real source of pleasure to me. In addition, Lynn had hoped that a strong male figure might help contain my behavior which was often bizarre or aggressive, having been affected by the combination of chemo and steroids. To the extent to which anyone could have made any difference, Nickie's presence was larger than life and at the same time he was a tender and solicitous companion.

I began having difficulty eating. Sometimes, for days on end, all I wanted was bowls of mashed potatoes from Laurier Barbecue, a restaurant near our house. Everything else tasted like dry wood. Janna Georges, who had by now joined forces with her husband and Lynn in the formation of my own personal wellness brigade, became adept at trying to waken my taste buds. I managed to eat an Arabic village dish, lentils with cracked wheat accompanied by yogurt. It was necessary to maintain stamina during the rigors of the treatment. There was always a pot ready if I felt hunger pangs. Mostly I drank cranberry juice or hot tea with squeezed lemons.

Finally I could no longer tolerate the dinner invitations, and some people were hurt by my last minute cancellations.

It was during this time that some of the contradictions of my personality surfaced. If I was considered to be a man of boundless energy, I thought I had to live up to the image. Ultimately, of course, I could not, and this sent mixed signals to many people I cared about. I guessed I needed too much reinforcement but punished myself and others in the process.

During my time hooked up to the chemo machine, the doctors all checked in on a daily basis, but they weren't as communicative as I would have liked. Reading the charts and hmming noncommittally with downcast eyes and then leaving as quickly as they had come did not fill my need for reassurance. I was the patient, and they the masters of my destiny.

Dr. Peter Gruner, a stocky man with an inviting face that seemed to say, "I know about suffering," proved to be a most compassionate, God-fearing man who has undergone much personal trauma, having lost a son and wife within a short time span. Still, he too, was unable to answer the barrage of questions with which we faced him. We wanted concrete answers and like Dr. Paul Beliveau, he dealt with statistics. I happened to be one of them. What guarantees could he give that would reassure us? He was already all that he could be, a dedicated doctor, a man of science and a cheerfully encouraging and wonderful listener. I would admit now that he was also patient to a fault.

It was the nurses in that department who were the real angels of mercy. I do not believe I would have seen the treatment to the end without their reinforcement and encouragement. My mind is full of vivid remembrances of nurse Judy Montesano who talked to me and with me and practically inch-by-inch pulled me through each day's treatment. I couldn't begin to imagine the emotional drain of the on-going nurturing of patients who face the demons of torment and *dis-ease* with the knowledge that at times only they will be there to snatch the life in their charge from the clutches of death. How psychologically grueling it must be for these nurses to keep their patients positive throughout the course of the treatment. I could not understand how they could remain so upbeat in the face of such a terrible and potentially devastating illness. Knowing the odds were that many of their patients would ultimately die, the nurses were still there giving the hope and courage that human beings need to keep fighting.

Even the appointments' secretary, who had seemed at first to be a pretty tough cookie turned out to be an extraordinarily sensitive team member. As time passed, I realized that she had a truly difficult job monitoring all the suffering patients who came through her office, each with a ready story to tell and questions to ask. In fact, anyone wearing a uniform became an authority figure to whom the soul in need turned for answers.

Many of the patients who began receiving chemotherapy about the same time as myself lost the battle along the way, in spite of the support of their valiant caregivers. The nurses were sympathetic to the occupants of the several Oncology rooms, young and old alike, who were connected to their chemo-lifelines. They appreciated that each had a history, a family and expectations.

My only critical thought was that no one thought to anticipate or explain in depth the possible violent reaction to the treatment. I became, in a word, deranged. One moment I would be happy and pleasantly assertive; the next, lethargic and completely disoriented. At another time, my mood would be angry, grouchy, and downright mean, especially to those closest to me.

In what I felt were my good moments, I conducted parish business by fax and phone from my hospital bed, much to the chagrin of the nurses, as the chemo dripped through the pipeline in my chest. As might be expected, this was not what they had in mind for my recovery. So vehemently insistent was I that there must be business as usual, that no one wanted to say no to my requests. They later confided to me that in the absence of any game plan, they let me do any outrageous thing I wanted, including faxing flurries of instructions to my office. They realized that permitting me to do what I believed needed doing might be as important a factor in my recovery as the chemotherapy.

Sometimes one of the chaplains would march in smiling broadly saying, "Hi, Father Antony, having a good day?"

I wanted to shout, "No! I feel like crap. Why are you smiling when I feel so lousy?" It was often so irritating and grating on my nerves to see those plastic, synthetic expressions of good cheer, or so it seemed to me then. Other patients in the ward were resigned to this kind of religious superficiality, but I found it offensive. In its own way, I suppose it was no different than the lack of sensitivity of some of the doctors.

Prior to my own first hand experience as a practical pastor, I constantly spoke about the need for sensitivity training for medical students to improve their communication skills. Everyone, no matter what their stage or situation benefits from a kind look, direct eye contact, a caress and real dialogue. The dilemma of modern medicine is the emphasis on learning technical skills without the concurrent commitment to acquiring beneficial human skills.

Lest one forget, while the medical staff cares for the body for a specific duration, the pastor has the totality of life in his charge, including helping the family members cope. I am no stranger to death. The sense of loss when a patient dies is no less traumatic to a clergyman than a doctor. Openness, not emotional shielding, is more conducive to wholesome and holistic medical care.

It was, therefore, especially difficult for me at that time to see how emotionally distant were many of the doctors. Doctors I knew well would peep in on me and then suddenly vanish like phantoms. I questioned them months later about their behavior, and asked why they did not come in, sit down next to me. The responses I received astounded me, an amalgam of their comments would read something like this, "We have seen your pathology reports. You have been a major figure in our lives, but according to what we read, you were dead meat. We were unable to deal with your frailty, or to face your mortality. We did not want to loose you."

I was incredulous. These were stunning statements. Did they really not comprehend how much I needed reassurance? Many times over the years I had held parishioners or even close friends facing death in my arms. There were some whose connection to life support systems was in my care. It was I who had to make the decision when it was time. I had held many a friend in the throes of death and gently nudged him or her in to the next phase in the journey. In each case there was lightness and sweet relief as they breathed the eternal "Ah!" How could professionals be so emotionally truncated? What kind of walls had they constructed to protect their mighty selves? Is death viewed only as a failure? As the awful enemy?

> *Death be not proud, though some have called thee*
> *Mighty and dreadful, for thou art not so,*
> *For those whom thou think'st thou dost overthrow*
> *Die not, poor death, nor yet canst thou*
> *Kill me.*

> ~ John Donne, *Holy Sonnets X*

As the treatments followed one another, other residual effects gradually were added to the mood swings, loss of hair, rapid weight loss, bleeding gums, and cracked skin. The bottoms of my feet became raw, and it seemed that my whole physique altered. I looked eighty.

Despite all this discomfort, I would not accept staying in the hospital during chemo-week. I insisted on going home each day; I wanted to be in my own space, ostensibly to rest but if I was fooling anyone it was myself. I continued to pester people to meet with me.

Lynn recalls she would wake up at night (more than once) to my having whispered conversations with people in my bedroom. I had phoned friends while she slept and urged them to come over and see me. I needed them. Her irritation and that of my children increased as each day passed with the comings and goings of people from outside our inner family circle.

Privacy is very important to Lynn. She needed to replenish her own resources in tranquility which I interrupted by the intrusion of so many of my dear friends. In addition she wanted me to rest. Irrationally I refused to accept her reasons, and she and the children felt for a time that I pushed them aside and included outsiders in my intimacy.

Antony Gabriel

The course of the treatment and my response to it was uneven. There were times when I wanted to be surrounded by vast numbers, yet within a short time, would throw everyone out yelling, "Leave me alone!" I became like a petulant child, hurt and depressed.

One evening my eldest son David attempted to reach me. I rejected outright any claim he might have on me or my time. I asked him to leave the house. When he phoned later, I slammed the phone in his ear. The next day I found an angry letter from him which was an eye opener, very revealing of his feelings toward his father, an altogether unflattering picture reflected in his words to me. Once again, it was as if scales fell from my eyes. Were my actions so obviously diminishing to the family? For that brief moment I realized that I had gone berserk, losing control of my sensibilities. I tucked my ego back into place and after pondering the pain I had caused, sat down and wrote him a loving note that I dropped off in the middle of the night at his home.

He told me later, "Dad, 1993 saw an assault on your body, but for me it was an assault on my mind. Thank you, for a healing message which I did not expect." David, my 6'5" giant, at thirty was a serious, studious young man who had inherited my penchant for the academic world. Yet he was still a son who saw his father sink into an irrational state and he did not have the appropriate mechanism to handle the situation. He had simply reacted under the pressure.

My family wondered, if I was dying, how they could reconcile all those unresolvable issues, the baggage that families collect over time or in the maturation of the relationship between parent and child. Suddenly, my children saw that possibility being stripped away from them. They could not fathom what to do with a father who vacillated between sweeping mood swings while entangling all sorts of people outside the family in his most private life.

In desperation, David, began to research the protocol that I was being given and discovered buried in an arcane medical journal some interesting facts and statistics about the physical and psychological impact of the treatment I was undergoing. These preliminary studies showed the percentages of patients who survive, who die or commit suicide during the treatment or because of it, I can now say that there were times when I too contemplated suicide.[4]

There were times when I was so angry and dispirited that I contemplated various scenarios that might look accidental or natural so I could still be buried by the church as a priest. In the Orthodox Church, religious burial for suicides is not the norm for laymen let alone for a priest. Some mystical force frustrated the pull to ultimate darkness. In any case, my son found some of the rationale for my erratic behavior which no one had anticipated, and therefore, there had been no warning to the family as to what might be in store for all of us. David's information was crucial to our understanding the dynamics at work.

At this time, I began to write truth letters to anyone I felt should recognize some truth about themselves which I could see and they could not. I conjured up every possible offense from the past. I wanted to right every wrong! If the treatment were to be unsuccessful, I would, at least leave no loose threads dangling.

It was Lynn who bore the major brunt of the psychological blows that I unwittingly and sometimes quite wittingly inflicted. Close friends who came to assist her during my chemotherapy were often horrified at my behavior toward her.

Finally, midway through the chemotherapy, after my rejection of her attempts at tenderness and understanding, Lynn accepted an offer to work as a reporter at a small community newspaper in Vermont. She rotated with her parents in caring for me during the remaining months.

During the interim weeks they would take me back to Vermont and, if we were all lucky, I would regain some equilibrium. I was tormented and through some perverse reasoning wanted everyone close to me to be co-sufferers. Another 20/20 hindsight.

Infrequently, during the Spring months, Lynn would talk me into accompanying her on a field trip for the paper. Throughout I could feel her drawing on inner reserves to remain upbeat and cajole me into thinking positively or trying to make things fun, but in general I resisted most of her suggestions and efforts. I simply walled myself off and did not even try to enter into a meaningful dialogue with her.

I had started work on a book on church history years before, and had boxes of research documents stacked neatly in my basement office in Vermont. I thought I might work on this project now, but I lacked the ability to concentrate sufficiently to consign any logical thought to paper. In terms of writing, organizational skills and ability to focus had deserted me. My attention span was limited to watching the afternoon soaps, staring into space, or just plain dozing on and off. The only writing that I was capable of was jotting down my inner thoughts about whatever struck me at the moment. Rereading these jottings today, I understand how really disjointed and fractured was my reality.

The center of the soul is God
when the soul loves and understands
and enjoys God to its utmost capacity
it will have reached its deep center: God.

~St. John of the Cross, *16th Century*

All spirituality and mysticism has its roots in the inborn desire of every sentient being to reconnect with our divine origin. All spiritual paths offer one formula or another which leads us to this reconnection by worshipping and nurturing the growth of that which is divine within each of us. In so doing we are then able to see, connect with and nurture that which is divine in others. The goal being to see only divinity around us, and the knowledge that only that which is divine is real and all else is illusion. All paths have an outward expression of worship which affirms the divine truth. As an Orthodox priest I am accustomed to an outward expression of faith in the Liturgy and celebration of the Divine Word. That is why I believed so much in the therapeutic-healing, positive energy force of the sacred music cassettes I listened to non-stop on a daily basis.

For months, however, I had been absent from the outward expression of my faith. I felt a void in my life, in the lack of communion and community. The interaction between a priest and the congregation can have dynamic effects on all participants and I missed it all!

In any case, for some sense of inner justification, I also felt I had to poke my head into the Church to reassure the parishioners, as well as myself, that I was still there. Throughout this period, whether wisely or not, I found myself presiding over the funeral services of a number of the elders in the Church, parents and close relatives to the founding families of the parish. When I was in chemo week and tethered to tubes and beeping machines, obliged to remain relatively stationary, I sent personal messages to be read by my assistant. Otherwise, if called upon I celebrated and preached the homily. I did not go to the funeral home or to the cemetery.

After the funeral service there is usually a meal of mercy, most often in the fellowship hall, during which bread is broken and the meal shared by the family and close friends of the departed. I often tried to be present at these meals, but with my immune system compromised by the chemo it became too risky to be in close contact with large groups of people, many of whom would rush to greet me with the traditional three (left, right, left) kisses on the cheeks. Of course, the practice had to be discouraged lest I contract some roving bug. Some understood, many felt rejected. Ultimately I had to give up going.

My young assistant Father Peter Shportun was thrust into the pastor's hot seat when the news hit that I would be out of the picture for a while. For someone of my nature it was a hard pill to swallow to have someone else running *my* show, so from time to time, I looked over shoulders and nudged parish business forward.

During Eastern Orthodox Holy Week, Father Joseph Purpura, the National Youth Director, was engaged to assist my associate pastor to conduct the various Church services, celebrated to overflow crowds. When it was time for the first service even though it coincided with chemo week, I stubbornly insisted on being a part of the ritual. Holy Week, without me at St. George? Unthinkable! Not possible! Cannot happen! I would be there.

In spite of Lynn's protestations, and the pleas of Council members that I remain at home, and against medical advice, I showed up for Palm Sunday Services. At one point during that service there is an outdoor procession around the block. It was a cold spring day and my teeth were chattering. In the style of some sort of Secret Service detail, a few council members surrounded and captured me fully vested and hustled

Antony Gabriel

me into a waiting car and drove me home.

Okay! Okay, I thought. I'll just go from chemo to home to bed for the rest of the week. Except, I wanted very much to attend the Holy Wednesday Evening Anointing Service. Again Lynn relented, agreeing to drive me with the proviso that I sit in a pew like everyone else, which I did more or less. However, by Good Friday, I was literally beside myself. How could I stay home on Holy Friday? I paced, I implored, I bargained, I threatened, I pleaded. Finally, Lynn succumbed and started the blah-blah about my being weak and the other blah-blah about bundling up and sitting quietly and all I could think was, "I win, I win!"

Once in the Church, I decided I would preside over the richly visual service in front of the floral decorated Tomb of Christ. I could not read the looks on the faces of parishioners as they watched the spectacle of their priest con-celebrating the Holy Friday Lamentations, red-faced, wobbly, weak-kneed, chanting overly loud to compensate. People were barely breathing expecting me to keel over at any second.

Lynn's patience had finally worn thin, she had *had it*! She strode quietly to the altar, and spoke quietly but sternly, "Kenny (my given name), this is quite enough. We're going home." I offered no resistance. The expression on her face was sufficient. Since it was pouring rain, friends surrounded me with umbrellas and once again I got into a waiting car.

On St. George's Day, April 23, we celebrated the Vesper Paschal Liturgy. At the conclusion of the service I received a Governor General's Award for humanitarian work, which was presented by Senator Marcel Prud'homme. The Church was packed with the faithful. The women of the Church outdid themselves in preparing for the reception that followed. It was a wonderful way to take a break from the dreary hospital treatment.

Throughout the period of treatment I occasionally held meetings at my home to deal with matters that required my overseeing. One such was a series of meetings with a psychologist and other case workers to launch a project to offer counseling to parishioners of St. George. Called the Family Service Program, it fell under the umbrella of Societe des Benevoles de l'Eglise St. George. It was intended for people who were in psychological pain, people who were grieving or in dysfunctional relationships. The goals being to contribute to a reaffirmation of personhood, and to help those in need to accept the possibility of changing destructive behavioral patterns.

It was also important to keep to the schedule of my meetings with couples seeking to adopt children from Lebanon. One such couple stopped by my home the same time one of the leading physicians from Beirut, who was also part of that adoption program was visiting. After this propitious meeting, a month or so later, the couple returned following their trip to the Middle East, with their newborn, newly-adopted daughter, only to discover that they themselves would become natural parents. It was as if the grace of their adopting a child from overseas generated a child of their own. This happened to more than one couple.

> *Make a joyful noise to the LORD, all the lands!*
> *Serve the LORD with gladness!*
> *Come into his presence with singing!*
>
> *Know that the LORD is God!*
> *It is he that has made us, and we are his,*
> *We are his people, and the sheep of his pasture.*
>
> *Enter his gates with thanksgiving*
> *and his courts with praise!*
> *Give thanks to him, bless his name!*
> *For the LORD is good;*
> *his steadfast love endures for ever;*
> *and his faithfulness to all generations*

~ Psalms 100

Antony Gabriel

Although we had been giving updates on my progress to my mother, there was always plenty of positive spin. For some reason no one had been entirely forthcoming with my father about what I was going through. All he knew was that I wasn't well and had needed surgery.

One afternoon late in the Spring, I felt compelled to travel to Syracuse to visit my aged parents. It was a hot, sunny day when I arrived and I removed my shirt. When my eighty-five year old father took a look at my emaciated body with the wide incision, and the porto-cath protruding from my chest, tears welled up in his eyes. He held my eyes with his own as he asked, "You have cancer, don't you?" I nodded. He stared quietly for a while and then said, almost cheerily, "Well, look at me. I had cancer and I'm still kicking." That was the extent of our conversation on the subject.

My mother-hen mother quickly intervened, clucking her upbeat comments and the ever-ready, waiting to be served though, always, just-out-of-the-oven or off-the-stove-top Lebanese meal. Is that what they all do? Tell us to "Just eat and everything will be fine?" I had gone home to reassure and relieve my parents to whom we had never told the full story. Who got the reassurance, especially from my mother? I also saw clearly that we never have any real secrets from those whose love for us is greater than we can imagine. At fifty-three years of age, my mother's comforting still filled me the with same warmth it had all my life. It never leaves. Is this not the reason the Virgin mother plays such an important role in the East?

My father had come to North America from the Zahle, Lebanon. His family settled in Lachine, Quebec, joining clan members from Zahle and Baskinta in a pattern typical of the first generation of immigrants. The family name was changed from Gibran to Gabriel; that's how it translated from Arabic to French. At the age of nine my father was placed in kindergarten to learn English. He soon felt too old, too tall and too out of place to continue so he quit and went to work.

My mother Nettie (Sopp), and father were typical of their generational background. Their marriage was arranged by their families, as soon as mother graduated from high school, and rapidly

GABRIEL'S DRAGON

produced five children, four sons and a daughter. My father was entirely self-taught, and with my mother instilled three basic principles in us, faith, the importance of education and the value of an honorable name.

Eventually, the family settled in the United States, moving around from Fort Wayne, Indiana to Toledo, Ohio before settling in Syracuse, New York. Everywhere, relatives offered the comfort of family ties and help in finding jobs. In those days, families took care of each other.

My mother combined business acumen with a warehouse of common sense. It was she who energetically sought the goal of owning their own business. She saved her pennies having been a child of The Depression, and by the 1950s had accumulated enough to acquire the now famous Gabriel Corner Grocery Store.

Both my parents were beloved by the neighborhood children for their enormous kindness. They never charged the less fortunate food taxes, and gave away so much food that they were later penalized by the tax department when the New York sales tax did not match the inventory.

My father had a keen sense of humor and was known as the funny man with the broad smile. He loved the Church and had a particular fondness for the Blessed Virgin, to whom he referred as *l'Athra* in his native tongue and for *Mar Ilyas*, or St. Elias, with whom he held frequent conversations inbetween periods of yelling at us to clean up the store or to get busy making deliveries.

At night he could be found lip reading from his Bible. He was a man of many parts, a man's man, and interested in world affairs. He wanted his own children to do better than he did and saw education as the route. He was committed to the democratic system, and the opportunities which it offered. Each of his five children received a university education thanks to this firm conviction and the push from both parents.

Tall, strong and handsome, even in his winter years, most people considered my father excellent company. It was many years before he told me that he was related to several Archbishops of the Church, including Germanos, Victor and Philip. He liked to share memories but not to brag. He died on September 12, 1995, a few days short of my parents' 67th wedding anniversary. He had lived with cancer for some

Antony Gabriel

time. There was no sense of a struggle or fight. My father met the dread enemy, acknowledged its presence and said to himself in effect, "So it's there, so what? I'm here and I'm going to enjoy myself." I say that these were his words, in effect, because my father often favored the use of those words which are the same ones many working class new immigrants learn first in English. We were taught by my very proper mother to sometimes treat dad's words as a code to be descrambled before relaying any of his messages to the outside world.

When I returned to Montreal after this visit I had several chemotherapy treatments left. I had needed, yet had been unable to internalize what lessons the comfort of my parents carried for me. Unlike my father I was increasingly unsettled. The longer the treatments lasted, the more unsettled I seemed to be. There was still rage and despair, doubts and uncertainty veering to acceptance and acquiescence then back again.

The cycles of life and death continued their rhythm in the universal flow.

I vividly recall a young professional woman who came to Montreal from Lebanon to continue her research on the effects of certain chemicals on cancer and AIDS. Soon after her arrival it was discovered that she had brain cancer. At first when I visited her home just prior to my own illness, as I did with all parishioners, she would closet herself in her room, leaving me with her mother. She had turned inward. Working in the medical laboratories, she was clearly aware of the progression of her disease, and she was unable to deal with it at first.

Later, when she learned of my own plight, we became fast friends. We spoke the same language, belonged to similar societies. She had great difficulty reconciling herself to God. We talked frequently by phone and in person. She was my neighbor in Outremont and therefore, frequently accessible for brief personal chats. As her disease advanced and the treatments were no longer effective, she entered the palliative care unit at the Royal Victoria Hospital. In the beginning it was difficult going there, but I forced myself. We continued our private conversations, until she finally accepted Holy Communion. I chanted hymns in her native Arabic language and hearing them woke something profound in her. I shall never forget her radiant smile as we bade one another farewell. She died peacefully, shortly thereafter knowing she was taking the next step on her journey to reconnecting with her divine origin, her creator, her divine self, her God.

It became an imperative for me to seek out those who were stricken with cancer and to assist themselves in coming to terms with themselves and God, and likewise their families who are the silent martyrs. They must bear within their hearts the burden of witnessing their loved ones undergoing immense personal trauma. I felt that as God had thus far spared me, I had an authentic voice to speak about the disease from the inside, as a priest, friend and fellow sufferer. Without exception, after each unique encounter, I was told both verbally and with intensely expressive eyes, "I know you know, Abouna, (Father)."

I believed I had a mission and began to reach out, as ever, obsessively, to other cancer patients, or to anyone who might have had a fatal illness.

Antony Gabriel

Love is a great thing, a good above all others.
which alone makest every burden light.
Love is watchful, and whilst sleeping
still keeps watch; though fatigued
it is not weary; though pressed, it is not forced.

~ Thomas à Kempis, *14th Century*

CHAPTER EIGHT

Out of Control

My frenzied, obsessive state of behavior was something, which viewed retrospectively by any sane man, could only seem hideous. Anyone who has ever involuntarily recalled his/her behavior or words, as being totally an inappropriate or miserably unsatisfactory response to situation(s), will also recall the cringing feelings that accompany those moments. Those recollections that come with eyes squeezed tightly shut, a wince and a profound wish not to have been there. The naked emperor prancing around with confidence extraordinaire!

During this hideous period, which I recall with all the above mentioned discomfort, in addition to my family and office staff the other victim of my despair and frustration was my father-in-law, Nick Georges. I had always felt very close to him; certainly I owed him a great deal in so many ways. Perhaps, in some ways these feelings made it safe, possible for me to strike out at him. The twenty year difference in our ages was never apparent in our relationship. He was always proud of his priest son-in-law; always believed I could do just about anything. He had recently retired from the restaurant business, and as soon as he learned of my plight, drove or flew in from Arlington, Virginia every chemo week to be with me. I think, in a way he felt he had a mission to see me through my ordeal. He was young in spirit, full of zest and determination, and he became my constant companion for weeks at a time. The fact that every once in a while he took a week to go back home (or somewhere), probably saved him from being driven to distraction by my antics.

At some point I decided I needed a new car. Magid Tarabulsi drove me to a Toyota dealership and I bought a new car on the spot, sight unseen, no test drive. I told the salesman what I wanted and it was there in a day or two, I think.

Nick had urged me not to do anything major without giving it a bit of thought. He really didn't believe I should be driving at all, and most people would have agreed with him. O, ye of little faith! In any case, a few days after it was delivered, I smashed my new toy. Nick then tried to dissuade me from driving any more, period. He said that's what he'd come for and assured me that he was ready at any time to take me anywhere I wanted to go.

One afternoon, when Nick had driven me home from chemotherapy, instead of resting and laying low as I had been told would be best, and as I most usually had done, I decided to give everyone the slip and took off to go swimming. I parked the car, left it running with the keys locked inside, and went in to the pool. Full of steroids, I swam wild laps for about an hour, banging my head against the pool wall at the end of nearly every other lap. By the time I left the building an hour and a half later, dressed and badly bruised about the head and face, the car was covered with snow and out of gas. Again, Nick rescued me. Not normally a patient man, in fact, impatient, was one of the words his family invariably used in describing him, Nick was extraordinarily patient and tolerant of my behavior. I know now that I really pushed hard to test his limits, but Nick was pretty adept at sidestepping my pushes. One look at those twinkling eyes and the deep-dimpled, slightly gap-tooth grin let any one who met him know that Nick himself was no stranger to mischief and enjoyed the challenge of trying to keep one step ahead of me. He did his job well and we both had some wonderful belly laughs. Sometimes he looked the other way and let me win, but after the swimming pool thing, he took charge of the car keys.

After each day's treatment he took me on hour-long power walks to tire me enough to make me want to go to bed. He was in his seventies at the time and still quite capable of energizing himself enough to seize control of the situation. Intuitively, he never confronted me. An athlete as well as an avid sports enthusiast, he was aware of the effects of steroids, so he pushed me in a different direction: brisk walks on the picturesque hills of Outremont.

Nick, who had helped me so much with my battle, was found to have a fast growing, inoperable, malignant tumor in his lung, in August, 1995, two weeks before the death of my own father. He had been operated on for colon cancer and had thought he was clean for several years. Ironically he'd been with us at the time and gone to my doctors to see why he was having severe pain in the hip. Much later we learned that the original tumors which had invaded his colon years before, had long ago sent seeds to the other areas.

Since he had been with us when the gravity of his health situation was revealed, he opted to stay in Vermont where we would be his primary caregivers along with Janna and his sister, Bebe Massouh. Over the next few months a steady stream of Nick's favorite people came and went at various times. It was a bittersweet time for all of us, but I must admit there was much more laughter than could ever have been predicted under the circumstances. The collective mood of the loving family gathered to walk with him as far as possible in this world, transcended every experience I had ever known or imagined for such a situation. His final days with us were a marvelous mixture of his enjoyment of having absolute and immediate access, day and night to everyone he really cared about and the soul-nurturing view through the glass doors or from the gallery of Mount Mansfield framed by the blazing colors of Autumn. His wit got sharper, and he used it in various ways daily to describe his feelings, and even his fears. The icing on Nick's cake was that it was Baseball World Series time and in the days leading up to the championship series, as his physical strength waned, the satellite dish brought a baseball game into view whenever he wanted it. Finally, the young man who had been there when Lou Gehreig played his 2130th consecutive game for the New York Yankees, his last, in 1939,

Antony Gabriel

sat bundled in an afghan on a mild autumn evening 56 years later. He was watching television, the wonder of youth still bright in his eyes, as Cal Ripken, hometown hero for the Baltimore Orioles, broke that record. Love and beauty, laughter and baseball; Nick's world was as it should be.

When in Dr. Silverstein's office the next day the doctor asked him if there was anything he needed or wanted to know, Nick, who, as usual, knew the score, asked the Dr. Silverstein if the doctor thought Nick would be around to see the Cleveland Indians take the Atlanta Braves in the World Series.

"Could be," the doctor answered, "but no guarantees. On the other hand Nick, no guarantees for sure they will take the Braves or that any of us will … "

"Okay, that's enough," Nick interrupted, putting up a hand to silence the doctor. He didn't like what the doctor was saying about the Indians or himself. He wished he hadn't asked.

Later as he saw the Indians doing poorly he asked that the game not be on while he was awake and that he not be told the scores. He was continually apologetic about disturbing the normal routine of our Vermont lifestyle. He never understood how privileged we felt to have him with us and what a gift his presence was to all of us.

Not quite through wrestling with all my own demons at the time, I tried at times to avoid what I felt was the death watch surrounding my father-in-law. Having the same original cancer, I felt acutely anxious for him, and, I admit, for myself.

However, on the morning of October 30, Lynn phoned me in Montreal to relay the message Nick wanted me there.

"What's the matter with him," Nick had asked, "doesn't he know I'm dying?" I sped back to Vermont.

Stroking his hand and kissing his forehead, I told him, "Nick, your being with us has been like having a real treasure in our midst. I know you're tired and it's okay. You need to continue on your journey. We love you, but you need to go and it's okay." Tears streamed down his cheeks and within a few minutes, he quietly and peacefully left. He had waited to say good-by in his own way. Anyway, the Indians lost, big time, and he was outta here!

GABRIEL'S DRAGON

They are not dead who live in lives they leave behind.
For those whom they have blessed they live a life again.

~ From a book about President Franklin D. Roosevelt

For some reason, during this hellish period, I thought I needed to be constantly buying things, like the new car. I went on buying binges seemingly trying to buy-up everything in my wake; an estate oriental carpet we could ill afford, new clothes, cases of Scotch whisky. Whatever craving entered my mind I felt needed immediate satisfaction. There was a great rush to do it all now, no holds barred. Anyone close to me was subjected to my whims and imperious behavior.

With terrific satisfaction on one level, I surreptitiously behaved in ways I knew Lynn would find objectionable, while at the same time, part of me was angry with her for not condoning the behavior I would ordinarily find bizarre.

One spring afternoon, I cajoled a friend, Georgina Howick, into taking me biking, much to Nick's frustration and dismay. With Georgina and without her, I rode all over Montreal. The build-up of the steroids made me feel omnipotent. I was out of control! I would give Nick the slip, sneak the bike out and roam wherever I could, as much a danger to others as to myself. I seemed, yet again, to be rushing headlong into one calamity after another. Thanks be to heaven that foolish behavior always brings about its own end. The damage that I did to my system as a result of this senseless expenditure of precious energy proved more dangerous than the cancer.

After the fifth chemo session, Nick called Lynn and advised her to return and take me to Vermont at the end of the week. We had no sooner arrived in Vermont than I became so weak and feverish, that she phoned the hospital in Montreal and was told to bring me to emergency. On the return trip, she took the back roads which usually cut the time by half an hour. As we drove by one of the familiar landmarks the Country Pantry Restaurant, I asked her to please stop so I could use the washroom. In view of my weakened condition Lynn wanted to come in with me. *Was it her goal in life to completely emasculate*

Antony Gabriel

me? I snarled sufficiently to convince her that I was still capable of standing at a urinal without her help. When after too long a time, I still hadn't returned to the car, Lynn came in and found me sitting at the counter eating a hot dog and french fries. As I had spent the previous day vomiting and hollering about the pains in my stomach, to put it mildly, Lynn was displeased.

We arrived an hour later, a gurney was brought to the car and I was rolled into the emergency room at St. Mary's. I was bleeding internally and there was talk of emergency surgery. The doctors asked Lynn whether I had eaten in the past few hours, and I said I had not. Lynn told them I had eaten less than an hour ago. There she goes again, I thought. I was suffering, probably dying and my wife was still trying to rob me of my dignity by calling me a liar!

"I did not eat," I shouted, or I thought I shouted. It seemed to me that no one was paying attention to me. I was so miserable, and everything hurt, and great waves of nausea were rolling over me, and nobody was listening to me!

We had been warned that the period toward the end of the treatment could be the most difficult because of the cumulative effect of the chemo. My body was reacting violently; I had lost thirty pounds and was in considerable pain. The morphine pump was hooked up again. Not only was there a massive reaction to the treatment protocol, but I had recklessly depleted my meager resources.

Our godson, Jeffrey Ayoub was to be married in Ontario that weekend and we had looked forward to being there. The Intensive Care Unit had not been part of the plan. I remember looking through the tubes carrying fluids to and from my body, fingering the morphine pump and thinking that, "if we turned this thing up enough, maybe I could make it through the wedding service."

After a period of time, the length of which was somewhere between two and four days, depending on who you ask, I made it out of ICU and back to a private room and access to a telephone.

My first contact with the outside world that morning came through a phone call from my assistant informing that they were fielding calls at the church office dealing with a rumor that I had only a few days, at most, to live. With all the sensitivity of a brussel sprout, he added that if that were not the case, I really ought to call people and tell them. It's okay, I thought. He's either very young or brain dead to believe it's my responsibility, right now, to reassure people that I am not dying. Anyway, maybe I am.

The hospital staff claimed that over a thousand people paraded in and out visiting me during this stay. Drawing and painting became my new pastime. I plastered the walls with all sorts of primitive art that reflected my mood swings, and amused my visitors, many of whom removed them as remembrances. At least, I prefer to believe that's why they removed them.

So many people crowded into my hospital room, that instead of waiting to be pushed aside again, my family simply fled the hoards of faithful who came to catch a final glimpse of me. I might have asked what was going on, having no idea why they were all there. I don't remember any answers. It was a strange collection of people who came, from diverse backgrounds; they came and they came, non-stop. I was, I supposed, some sort of shrine.

One afternoon I awoke to a room filled with several people dressed in black, chanting in Arabic and crying. At the center was Myrna, a woman who is said to exude holy oil from her hands. She had been to church the Sunday after I'd completed my fifth chemo cycle, just prior to my marathon biking expeditions. When I saw this motley crew hovering at my bedside, I thought, with no small hint of relief, that I was perhaps really dead. Someone of them was touching my hands saying, "We will never forget you." Weakly, I waved them out while screaming to Myrna in my head, "You and those oil-leaking hands cannot save me. Get out!"

Others came and I launched, again, into tirades settling any long-standing disagreements I felt existed. I remember asking as I watched visitors come and go, "Have they no mercy? They're so obvious, coming because I'm dying."

I was unable for a time to swallow anything solid, so I put out requests for popsicles. In a few days the staff ordered a halt. Every freezer in the wing was overloaded. They had to distribute popsicles

Antony Gabriel

throughout the hospital. It was June, there was an electricity brownout, it was hot and there was a flood (of sorts) when they melted.

I shocked my young secretary, Stephanie, when I called her one day asking her to bring me strawberry flavored condoms. To this day I do not know why I did so. An earlier prostate operation removed any need of my use for condoms and in any case I was certainly in no condition to need one.

What I did *not* know at the time was that I was in the palliative care unit and that my presence was causing inappropriate commotion. The nursing staff complained that the endless procession of visitors was disturbing to the other patients.

On St. Jean Baptiste Day, June 24, we traditionally celebrate our dear friend Cookie Rossy's birthday. In general, there is a small group of us who celebrate June-July birthdays with a series of meals and parties. I did not want to miss this one. I signed myself out, telling the nurses I was just going home for a bit. I didn't have the nerve to say I wanted to go to a party. I called my son Mark to drive me home saying I just wanted to be in my own bed for a while. I said I would sleep a bit and call him later to take me back. I did sleep with a wonderful sense of relief after Mark left. However, instead of calling him when I awoke, I drove myself the four miles or so to the Rossy's home for the party. Before I had been there ten minutes I was shivering, despite the heat of the day. I started reeling and felt tossed about in a huge sea of nausea. Mercifully, my host came to my rescue and drove me back to St. Mary's, where I belonged and should never have left in the first place.

Back in my hospital bed, feeling defeated I think I apologized on an average of every five minutes for the rest of the day, for having caused so much disruption, still not realizing that I was the one I had most disrupted. Doctors and nurses invented some new language in chastening me and there was little if any sympathy. This time they were stern and angry and rightfully disgusted at my behavior. I was told in terms used to explain to first grade children that I was in a crisis, which for the most part, I had precipitated; that I was to stay put, and that my phone was being disconnected. That was okay with me, I was tired and needed to rest. Why did they have to be so snappy, so harsh!

That harshness, as it turned out, had to do with the fact that the staff was fed up with me and so many of mine. During my absence, some parishioners had used the St. Jean Baptiste Holiday to come and visit me and found my bed empty. When they asked one of the nurses where I was, she apparently threw out a backhanded wave and without looking up said, "He's gone!" To them it meant I was dead.

By the next day the Church office began receiving telephone calls requesting the times of visitation at the funeral home and funeral services. The office also had to field questions from the press, including a request for an official statement.

I now understand that the part of me that knew I was gradually slipping away was grasping at anything to assure myself that I was still alive. The oncologist later confided that I was, indeed, on the edge of the abyss during those June days. It came as no surprise to me.

After several weeks of suspended existence and morphine dreams, I was ready to go home. I knew I would thrive in my own space. The hospital had become an alien hostel and I wanted out! I was released on a Saturday afternoon in an emaciated condition. My sons carried me to my bedroom.

Dispirited, I floated in and out of consciousness. The medication, I believe, had a profound impact on my will and my perceptions. There was a pervasive medicinal odor wafting around me. Looking in the bedroom mirror, I saw a caricature of my former self. It was terrifying. The awful smell was everywhere! There was an ugly porcupine/skunk inside my head firing quills of odious, foul, smelling emanations in all directions. I prayed for the nausea to abate. Placing a cushy down pillow between my bony knees, I used the last of my remaining energy to draw myself into a fetal position and hoped it wouldn't be too long before someone came to dry my tears and wipe my nose.

Antony Gabriel

So every faithful heart shall pray to thee in the hour of Anxiety, when great floods threaten. Thou art a refuge to me in distress so that it it cannot touch me; Thou dost guard me in salvation beyond all reach of harm.

~ Psalms 32

CHAPTER NINE

The Turning Point

On Sunday morning, I was awakened to the sound of the telephone ringing on the first floor. Lynn brought the receiver to me. "It's for you," she said, grinning with the knowledge that I would relish the call. It was my granddaughter, Caitlin. "Hi, Poppy," she said enthusiastically, it's my birthday! Are you coming over? You're not going to miss my party, are you?"

"Absolutely not," I said in a voice so strong I startled myself, "I'll be there soon!"

It was as if that small voice was my connection back to life. To have disappointed her would be unthinkable. At the same moment the decision to go to her birthday party was made, I felt a tiny, inexplicable jolt of strength enter my body. I had to go.

Too weak to shout, I used one of the two telephone lines to phone Lynn on the other. She had been preparing breakfast and was caught off guard by the announcement that I would need help to get dressed for Caitlin's party. I remember very little of the day, except watching Caitlin's excitement at having both sets of grandparents there for her special day. I am left with the one delightful image of that innocent face beaming with self-conscious pleasure at her good fortune; her glances darting between her loved ones and the stack of presents waiting to be opened.

In my weakened condition I wasn't able to stay long, but the effort resulted in such a rush of pleasure that I knew recovery was a sure thing. We drove to Vermont where I could shore up strength for the sixth and final cycle of the treatment protocol.

Lynn, too, seemed to have picked up on the subtle change that had come about since my phone conversation with Caitlin that morning. The drive to the country was leisurely and peaceful for the first time in many months. Conversation, although sparse, was easy and totally devoid of tension. There was the quiet acknowledgment between Lynn and I that a new peace and sense of wellness had been born. The next few days became extended moments of solemnity which were at the same time, bursting with an indescribable joy that bordered on giddiness.

It was Springtime and I actually saw it coming. In a matter of days, I watched through the living room window, as through some time-lapse photo lens, as Mount Mansfield turned a tender green.

While drinking my morning tea on the balcony, I called excitedly for Lynn to observe with me the two hummingbirds trying to push their way through the glass doors of the bedroom. Hummingbirds actually hover in mid-air. How can they just hang there? Lynn was writing on deadline and answered laughingly that it was an observation that we'd made every year since we'd first come to Vermont. She was mightily mistaken. I thought I had never seen anything so amazing in my entire life. The brilliant sun shone like God's own glory in this bucolic setting and every instant gave another nuance of shade to the color green. Another first awakening.

> Brothers have no fear of men's sins.
> Love a man even in his sin, for that
> is the semblance of Divine Love
> and is the highest love on earth.
> Love all God's creation, the whole
> and every grain of sand in it.
> Love every leaf, every ray of God's
> light. Love the animals, love the plants,
> love everything.

GABRIEL'S DRAGON

*If you love everything, you perceive
the divine mystery in things. Once
you perceive it, you will begin to
comprehend it better every day. And
you will come at last to love the
whole world with an all embracing love.*

~ Theodore Dostoevsky, *Brothers Karamazov*

One of the most difficult aspects of any process in facing one's own imminent mortality is relating to family and friends. It is a time when the patient seeks one or several persons in whom to place confidence and trust. Although several may reach out to help, the person engaged in the life and death struggle cannot easily deal with many personalities in this orbit which culls and restricts itself.

Often a friend or loved one is deeply hurt or offended when emotional support genuinely offered is summarily rejected. It is important that any member of a support system be aware that his or her role will vary greatly from time to time. The emotional stability of the patient will be in flux and decisions as to who is the chosen one of the moment may seem arbitrary and, in fact, may be so. The toxic nature of treatment protocols and of the illness itself wreak mischief and considerable havoc with the mind and body.

It is an incredible blessing and facilitator of wholeness to have a caring support system of family, close friends and people whose strength is ready when needed, and who can accept being thrust aside for no apparent reason.

My granddaughter Caitlin was a very special lifeline. In her own way, she retrieved me from the edge. Perhaps more specifically it was my love for her and a reverence for the faith and trust which she represented as a simple matter of fact. My relationship with Caitlin is and was very simple and uncomplicated. This provided a great relief in the midst of all the other complications I was feeling. She loved me, and I could feel that. She had complete faith in my recovery and I could feel that. With all the innocence of childhood, whenever Caitlin was in my

Antony Gabriel

presence, she looked after and encouraged me in a way both childlike and strangely mature.

I continued to experience a lot of discomfort and cracking of the skin on the soles of my feet as one of the side effects of the chemo. One weekend when Caitlin was staying with us, she noticed my feet propped up on pillows. My immediate impulse was to throw a cover over them to protect her from having to look at the exposed fissures, and to protect my own sensitivity to what I was sure would result in her revulsion. Instead, her facial expression reflected an empathetic pain. "Ooh, Poppy, poor you," she cried, "these must hurt you so much! I really should anoint them for you!" She actually used the word anoint.

With every confidence that she was doing what needed to be done, she went into the bathroom and returned with the proper medicated cream (I could only suppose that she'd seen Lynn use it at some earlier time). She then proceeded to sit on the bed and, wordlessly, placing my feet in her lap, began rubbing the cream into them, gravely studying her task. I watched in awe wanting to both laugh and cry as I saw her purse her lips and shake her head from time to time. When the mission had been completed to her satisfaction, she tucked my feet under the covers and patted them twice. "I think I healed you a little, Poppy. You'll be just fine, now," she said with an air of authority. I believed her; she was four years old and I believed she knew what she was saying. Her look and gesture is indelibly etched on my heart.

On another occasion Caitlin was spending the night with us and we watched a television news program on which I had been filmed making hospital rounds shortly after a chemotherapy session. During the interview, I had made reference to her importance to my healing process. Stretched out on the bed between Lynn and me, when Caitlin heard my reference to her she buried her head in her hands and said, "Oh, Poppy, are we ever famous now!"

There is a love like a small lamp, which goes out when the oil is consumed; or like a stream, which dries up when it doesn't rain. But there is a love that is like a mighty spring gushing up out of the earth; it keeps flowing forever, and is inexhaustible.

~ Isaac of Nineveh, *7th Century*

Antony Gabriel

CHAPTER TEN

Celebration, Faith and Community

I feel God is traveling
so much in me, with the dark and the sea.
With Him we go along together. It is getting dark.
With Him we get dark. All orphans …

But I feel God. And it even seems
that He sets aside some good color for me.
He is kind and sad, like those who care for the sick;
He whispers with sweet contempt like a lover's:
His heart must give Him great pain.

~ "God" (Dios) in Neruda and Vallejo

To celebrate my last chemotherapy treatment, my cousin George Saba, his wife Janice and their four children hosted a birthday party for me in mid-July, a few short weeks after my having nearly checked out of this earthly existence. Many of our parish friends were invited and encouraged to bring gag gifts. I was thin as a rail, and nearly bald except for a few sporadic patches of white fluff here and there.

In spite of my frail state, I wanted to do the driving for the ten miles or so to their home. In an effort to avoid a confrontation with my father-in-law over who would drive, I convinced him that since I knew the way it would be easier for me. I also promised that if I felt the least bit weak, I would give him the wheel. By now Nick was a master at walking the tightrope of balance between watching out for me and still allowing me some face-saving independence. By the time we arrived we both knew I shouldn't have been behind the wheel. I was no better than a drunk driver and we had both been irresponsible.

I was absorbed enough in myself that I was able to enjoy the party, even though I knew Nick was nervous thinking I might want to drive home against our mutual better judgment. In any case, his mind was made up and throughout the evening while others laughed and celebrated, Nick (as he later informed me) thought only of his resolve that there would be no repeat performance on the ride back. He maintained that his own self-absorption with the instinct to survive had taken over. According to Nick, to keep his heart and stomach in their proper positions and functioning normally, meant he would, again, have to put his foot down – on the gas pedal this time. Sorry, Big Nick, I sure gave you a rough time!

At about this time it became a compelling personal mission to share my own unique experience with stricken parishioners, friends, mere acquaintances, and often any stranger of whose travail I might inadvertently learn. To say that I was obsessed would be a gross understatement. I was looking for cancer patients! I sought out cancer patients! From the hospital and while at home, barely able to function, myself, I got their telephone numbers and addresses. If I felt more was needed, I visited them in their homes or in the oncology units. I wanted the patients to draw positively on their own inner resources. I believed that even in the more advanced stages, the quality of life can be continually improved and my message on retraining thinking and outlook needed to be told.

While I could not possibly sustain to this day the sense of urgency I felt at that time to pass on that message, I still believe it is an important one.

Courage and hope for patients and their families as they confronted

Antony Gabriel

together the various stages of cancer became our link. We prayed together, read the scriptures, especially the Psalms and the Gospel stories and talked openly about their feelings. A bond was created by the fact that we all shared the same illness.

The physicians who were aware of my activities thought it absolutely ludicrous for me to undertake such work since I was myself not out of the woods. Nevertheless, I believed that since we are all a part of the human family, to which we have divine responsibilities, it fell to me to spread the message to my co-sufferers.

During my pastorate I had spent many hours in cancer counseling. The notion that any insight I'd gained from having a blood disease gave me the inside track on suffering turned out to be a superficial assumption. While it may not be entirely fair to those among us who do feel genuinely the pain of their loved ones, I was sure at the time that one never truly understands much of anything without the existential experience.

In a moment of crisis, there comes that awesome realization that nobody promised us a rose garden. God gave us one in the very beginning of things. All we had to do was to tend it and follow a simple rule. When we did not, we had to leave; our own free will makes choices daily which bring us future blessings or burdens. Still, even outside the garden God walks with us as he did with Abraham. He is faithful in helping us bear our burdens.

True faith never justifies sickness and death as part of God's plan for humanity; man was created with perfection the goal of a loving God. Humanity has separated from the communion with God by rejecting His will. Still there are bright moments in history when our will intersects with His and blind moments when it does not.

Separated from God, man has become infected with sin, and vulnerable to disease and therefore death. To use the graphic expression of C.S. Lewis, man became bent.

God offered the gifts of life, love and freedom. He does not inflict punishment on his children by sending disease, war or death. Our life-styles (choices) may, but certainly not God. I am not a medical doctor, but experience has led me to the belief that there are many complex factors involved in our illnesses. Heredity, our personal destructive behavioral patterns, the eroding environment, stress, and the foods we eat all play their own role.

Since disease and death are part of the human dilemma, what is important to our survival and its quality is how we deal with these realities. Blaming or ascribing to God all our calamities does us no good. That train of thought reduces God to punisher and denies human responsibility for any situation.

Christians believe in creative suffering through which a person is reborn through cycles of pain, death and rebirth. Man suffers to be regenerated; man dies in order to be reborn, to be transformed into a new existence.

The texture of human existence is imbued with the rhythm of life, death and rebirth; suffering death and resurrection. These are not only Biblical themes. They are also the themes of great literature and philosophical reflection. "Who am I? Why am I here? Where am I going?" are questions asked by poets, prophets and truth seekers throughout the ages.

Death is not a failure, not the end, but the beginning of a wondrous rebirth. It seems to me that what makes death so fearsome is the inability to love. Not to fulfill one's potential, not to do some good in this life is death already while we are alive. Physical death, after a fruitful, productive life is but a phase, a transition to the only true reality. In a way, life is but a preface to eternity.

> *Cowards die many times before their deaths;*
> *The valiant never taste of death but once.*
> *Of all the wonders that I have yet heard,*
> *It seems to me most strange that men should fear,*
> *Seeing that death, a necessary end,*
> *will come when it will come.*

> ~ William Shakespeare,
> *Julius Caesar, Act II, Scene II*

Antony Gabriel

In counseling others my main purpose is to help the co-sufferers dig deep within themselves to rediscover the spark of God which is within each of us. This quest for God is, in itself, a healing agent. However, when the time for the transition to eternity arrives, a true healing means that it can be embraced with courage and faith. No one can stay forever in this earthly plane. When our mission on earth is completed, there is no terror, but peace when one releases the spirit to the Giver of all life. The peace that surpasses all human understanding floats the spirit to a new region of being.

This brings to mind the example of Father Jean Meyendorf, a world famous Byzantine theologian, professor and recently retired Dean of St. Vladimir's Seminary in New York. In his mid-sixties, he was looking forward vigorously to more productive years of writing and adding to an already prodigious literary output.

A few months prior to my own encounter with cancer, I received a startling call from St. Mary's Hospital telling me that Father Jean was critical and asking for me. He had been taken to the hospital from his summer retreat in the Russian colony at Labelle, Quebec. I rushed to the hospital where I joined his valiant wife Micka and children at the bedside vigil. He was dying of pancreatic cancer that had gone undetected until the previous week.

He was my priestly role model, the sponsor at my ordination and the one other person besides Dr. Arthur Vööbus who had believed in whatever intellectual skills I had to pursue graduate studies. I was shaken to the core at the prospect of losing such a cherished friend.

We spoke on a daily basis, and our conversations covered many subjects. It was as though he had to get things off his chest. There was an urgency in his heavy breathing as he struggled to say it all.

Towards the end, with amazing lucidity and with such serenity as I had never imagined possible, he looked at me and said, "You know, Antony, I retired and bought a home near Yale. I thought I would be finishing several more books on Byzantine history, theology and patristics; they're all in my head." Then he shrugged his shoulders, made a whooshing sound through puffed out cheeks, and with a wry smile said, "Ce que l'homme propose, le bon Dieu dispose." (What man proposes, the Good Lord disposes.)

Father Jean taught a concept in his classes, drawn from all the known ancient sources that he uncovered for us: Synergy, co-operating with God. This is a courageous act. Synergy means, in lay jargon, our will being open to God's will for us. It implies the unfolding of our heart to that higher reality that empowers us to qualitatively live better or to accept the call to the kingdom. Our energy/will connects to the energy/will of God Himself. That is Grace.

In later months, during long periods of self-examination, his image reappeared on numerous occasion and what it brought to mind was the word "courage," the same word Mother Theresa used to sign her correspondence. Father Jean's submission to God was a sign of his courage.

How often have sufferers wrestled with or rejected God altogether in the throes of distress? Too often the early memories of our childhood relationship with God fades with the vicissitudes of life and time. Our souls and hearts become encrusted. Once we stand face to face with the awful consequences on diseased bodies, we shrivel at the prospect of sustaining a lengthy illness and at the same time fill with dread at our pending demise.

A mental decision must be made for life, to plug willingly into that ultimate life force, the Source of limitless energy and grace. Sickness can re-sensitize us to ourselves, to the inner self that has been lost in the maze of life's undertakings.

> *In all events of life, however untoward they may be,*
> *the wise man encourages us to rejoice instead of*
> *giving way to sadness.*
> *In so doing, we will not loose the greater good, peace*
> *of mind in both prosperity and adversity.*
>
> ~ St. John of the Cross, *16th Century*

Antony Gabriel

As a postscript to this section, I would like to add that from the earliest days of my priesthood I have been in awe of death. Today, this sentiment is even more profound. The mystery of death is probably the most elusive question and profound paradox of life man deals with. Most people try to avoid even thinking about dying. For a member of the clergy, constant contact with the dying and death, makes it an inescapable daily reality. Just as the reality of sickness cannot be sanitized (nor should it be) death cannot be plasticized nor cosmetically beautified. Neither can it be wished away. At the bedside of a dying person, one can but bow the head in reverence as the person is ushered into eternity. Over the years, I have clasped many a dying person's hands as the tears rolled down his or her cheeks during a tender prayer. Then suddenly the eyes open wide as though seeing a powerful vision and he or she breathes a momentary "Ah!" as the spirit leaves the body. The tears of those departing are the sign of their final farewell.

The crossing of the thin dividing line between two worlds is amazing to witness. In one instant the walls of the house crumble, and "whoosh," the spirit has gone to a new dimension. This was exactly what happened at the bedside of my father-in-law, Nick. Seldom have I experienced anything less than light and peace at such a scene.

To this day, presiding over a funeral, I can but kneel before the awesome specter of death. It's very existence makes each day even more precious. *Time* is the one gift of God that we can return to him freely in loving, giving and serving. One sage remarked that the man of faith who thinks that this day will be his last, will surely live more completely, conscious of his actions.

The principle thing is to stand
before God with the mind in the heart,
and go on standing before Him
unceasingly day and night, until the end of life.

~ St. Theophon the Recluse

GABRIEL'S DRAGON

CHAPTER ELEVEN

The Enigma of Life

───────────

When on the road to Thebes,
Oedipus met the Sphinx,
who asked him her riddle,
his answer was: Man. This
simple word destroyed the monster.
We have many monsters to destroy.
Let us think of Oedipus' answer.

~ George Seferis
Speech upon receiving the Nobel Prize
(1967)

In the search for meaning, the so-called traditional modality in the West has come to a dead end. The people who are out there dealing with life and death issues want answers.

The aberrations in the churches are poignant reminders of their lack of depth. At Christmas, the minister at a Protestant church presented a puppet show instead of a homily on the nativity. During the Pope's last visit to Montreal, there was a ballet danced by a priest carrying the Gospel during the Papal Mass.

Neither affluence, science nor technology adequately responds to the inner hunger for divinity, and certainly not play acting during a church service in the name of relevance. Contemporary man, society, religion and life itself, have all been stripped of mystery. The *mysterium tremendum* of God is no longer. The words of the prophets, Jesus, the miracle stories, the resurrection have all fallen under the intellectual microscope of today's so-called scholars who have relegated them to the status of mythological. In other words, they are not truths for men to live by.

Hence, the rise of interest in the spirit world; angels, faith healers and gurus, all of whom have displaced God. Throughout the ages, men and women have sought satisfactory answers to the ultimate questions of birth, life, illness and death.

For the East, the mystery of the mystical abides. There are no neat divisions. The bridge is crossed by Jesus. The Christ of faith and the Jesus of history are One. In worship we no longer see "... looking through a glass, darkly," and all is made clear in that ineffable encounter with the Lord of All. Yes, angels are fundamental to scriptural belief, but so too are the miracles of divine intervention in history.

Perhaps a little more humility is required in discussing the nature of God and his revelations. The Biblical proclamation and symbols ought to be viewed as a loving message from another world that is beyond all our relativistic categorization. Maybe we need to transfer our gaze to the world of eternity and focus less on the temporal world.

We have been created in His image and likeness, but in the arrogance of our era, we have reversed this by re-fashioning him according to our phenomena.

Our youth-oriented society has worked strenuously to erase the reality of suffering; redemptive suffering and most certainly death has been embalmed. The logical conclusion of godlessness in the face of death is despair. Atheism, empiricism and materialism have no message for the dying and the weeping.

I am an image of Thy glory ineffable, though I bear the brands of transgressions: show Thy compassion upon Thy creature, O Master, and purify me by Thy loving kindness; and grant unto me the home-country of my heart's desire, making me again a citizen of paradise.

~ Orthodox Funeral Service

At the time of my illness, I think I was too numb to take death into account; therefore, I was not afraid of death itself. Even though I heard the words of mortality, and three times was almost swept away, the fear of its awesome power somehow eluded me. To this day, I do not know why. Quite probably I subsumed this thought in the subterranean of consciousness. While I do not dwell on it, my senses are more attuned to death today.

During the last period of chemotherapy, when death's immanence was most present, there was an overriding theme to my thoughts. Here, for fear of being trite, I will tread cautiously through the delicate terrain.

Something stirred deep inside of me saying that the ego gratification of the past must be gone forever. A priest has no mission to jettison himself or his message from the pinnacle of personal power. I felt I had to give voice to a different, perhaps a whole new dimension of faith and practical spirituality in a secularized society. I felt I had to be a wounded healer for others. In the words of St. John of the Cross I had " ... a wound that is a gift."

I recalled hearing Caitlin's little voice that had jolted me out of death's jaws during the past weeks of treatment. It provoked even more profound contemplation as I meditated in the quiet of my study at home, the walls covered with ancient, precious icons. This room is my small paradise or kingdom; a sacred space. There is, for me, an almost palpable spiritual energy in that study filled with icons and books.

Rhythmic prayer took on a life of its own, deep within. I trained my breathing to coincide with personal prayer so it would move freely and carry me on its wings. Either sitting in the study, or lying in bed with eyes shut, or focused on a favorite icon, I let the prayer do its work.

Antony Gabriel

Chanting the Jesus prayer,[5] a verse from the Psalms, or any sacred scripture, or some form of the Divine Name is a time-tested method for centering and establishing a norm for daily meditation.

In the act of prayer and meditation, one must always bear in mind that one does not and cannot stand before God as a beggar. That would make the worshiper nothing more than a slave. Prayer is not a bargaining tool. It is a source of communion with all being. Through prayer and contemplation, one creates a store of divine energy that sustains us in the midst of pain and suffering. It can be said that holiness is yearning made manifest.

> *When we trust God with our whole heart, we don't fill our prayers with "Give me this or take this from me." We don't even think of ourselves when we pray. At every moment we trust our Father in heaven, whose infinitely surpasses the love of all earthly fathers and who gives us more than we ourselves could ask for or even imagine.*
>
> ~ Isaac of Nineveh, *7th Century*

While it was a struggle at first, meditation soon became a part of my daily routine, without which I could not manage the daily threat of death. I reflected often on the peculiar ability of some people to remain closed in on themselves as they passed through the dark night of the soul, confronting catastrophic illnesses. Stillness can bring a voice of its own, as one mystic wrote, "Silence is the language of the Kingdom."

Years ago I attended a banquet given in honor of Pope Shenouda of the Coptic Church in Egypt. It was a testimonial to this bishop of the Church who had only recently been released from years of house arrest by the Egyptian civil authorities.

Hundreds were in attendance, anticipating a message from this courageous Christian witness. However, when he entered the large hall, he blessed the assembly in absolute silence and left as the crowd watched in silence. It took me a long time to realize that his silence spoke louder than words. He was, after all, the heir to a long lineage of Egyptian desert fathers who sat in silence for years. He authenticated his suffering through silence, that is, he gave God his pain and communicated to us redemption and victory: "If he is not edified by my silence, there is no hope that he will be edified by my words." (Pambo)

Humor is a prelude to faith,
and laughter is the beginning of prayer.

~ Reinhold Niebhur

Laughter is, of course, another vital element of survival. While much has been written recently concerning the mechanism of laughter and it's effects on our well being, I felt I had rediscovered that reality. There are times when we are so miserable and frustrated with our own situation that we can barely communicate our needs or feelings to those who might be able to help. Laughing at oneself is a tonic against depression. Once laughter diffuses a tense, painful or fearful moment, we are better able to see that moment clearly. Maintaining a sense of humor is a key component in dealing with the vicissitudes of daily life, not to mention a life threatening disease. Easier said than done, perhaps, but every available tool must be used to transform fear and self-doubt to an affirmation of life.

Lynn and our close friends brought many of my favorite videos and we were entertained by the antics of Peter Sellers, and some classic Charlie Chaplain. Hilarity is a marvelous way to rekindle the joie de vivre. The antidote to sullenness is joy. Levity alters the body's alchemy while uplifting the spirit and helping to float away pain.

Swimming was also a wonderful relaxation for me as well as a way to maintain or regain strength. Whenever I entered the water I was able to shed any worries or preoccupations I was carrying at the moment.

Antony Gabriel

Swimming also allowed me to feel healed; whole. Some of the most fortifying insights came to me as I swam. Perhaps it was the combination of breathing and rhythmic prayer, the feeling of being held safe and some coincidence of openness on my part to the occasional beauty of a sunbeam sparkling on the water. Swimming gave me a temporary respite and allowed a space for my thoughts to come together again. As I stroked or floated in the water, ideas for my daily journal and ultimately for this book took shape.

I listened and read every conceivable self-help book and tape that fell into my hands. Most were in one way or another useful to me in providing valuable insights to dealing with the cancer. They were meaningful sign posts for the inward journey. In reality, every positive effort we make or discover for ourselves has a good return when dealing with a life-threatening disease, and there is always a time when the message or experience of others touches us, if we allow it.

Later I was struck by the fact that so many modern psychologists and psychiatrists (at least the ones who write books) use Greek mythology as paradigms for modern relationships.[6]

The contribution of music to my return to wholeness cannot be overstated. I even slept with music. The earphones were plugged in to the portable cassette player and stayed with me throughout the night. Who knows what impact the flow of beautiful uplifting music has on one's deepest subconscious?

Listening to sacred chants the miracle that awakened in me was not only that of giving myself over to the Lord, but at the same time, an awareness that in most ways, my life was still in my own hands. No matter what kind of support system or medicine or mechanism, I still had to do it myself! It was up to me to seize control of my own destiny and not to succumb to blind fate.

I came to see disease as a kind of separation, a process of fragmentation and disintegration that I had to halt by the reintegration of my spirit with my body. Losing my ego (still working on it) and discovering the God within was the ultimate task and challenge that confronted me. Prayer and meditation, swimming, laughter and the stacks of self-help books and tapes were just tools and vehicles along the way.

GABRIEL'S DRAGON

It was not the loss of the body that provoked me to action, but the lessons learned in suffering; to regain a sense of purpose and responsibility to myself and others. I had been made aware that I would be leaving too much unfinished personal business if I gave up, as I had at times been tempted to do.

> *When your life is filled with the desire to see the holiness in everyday life, something magical happens: ordinary life becomes extraordinary, and the very process of life begins to nourish your soul!*

~ Rabbi Harold Kushner

Antony Gabriel

CHAPTER TWELVE

The Struggle Between Life and Death

... there fell from his eyes as it had been scales ...

~ Acts 9:18

All this philosophical reflection and the conclusion may sound easy but it in fact it was not. This was a struggle between life and death in the full sense of the word. Long buried sins, past mistakes, tensions, scars of old wounds, broken relationships all came to the surface along with life's many blessings. There is no more humbling experience that the face-to-face encounter with the prospect of imminent mortality.

"Everything happens for a reason," was the recurring theme in the justification of my crisis. The illness brought with it a sharper than ever-before spiritual awareness.

It became startlingly apparent that a form of real messianic complex had played itself out in my life and ministry. My values, my moves and my motivations stood before me in bold relief; they were no longer the rock upon which a life could be built.

I felt like the child in C.S. Lewis's, *The Boy Who Became a Dragon*. When the hard scales were ripped off the Lion (the supreme loving authority in that tale), he suffered unspeakable pain when his sins were pulled off like artichoke leaves to reveal the persona at the core he had been trying to conceal. There was no corner of my life left unexamined. However, a decision had to be made within: Forget the past accept the present, to meet each challenge, and to strive always to conquer temptation in its many subtle forms.

For some unknown reason the figures of my grandmothers, Anna Sopp and Nazleh Gabriel,[7] re-emerged vividly in my consciousness at this time. Their lives, their history and words helped shape my youth, and their candor and wisdom propelled me forward as I strove to become a priest. Their presence in our lives also helped me to appreciate the wit and wisdom of our elders and what they impart to us through steadfast character. Now, once again, their example of endurance and unswerving faith in the face of great odds loomed before me. They were my "Lion." I thank God for their presence as I look back at this period of my life.

> *Man is born to live, not to prepare for life.*
> *Life itself, the phenomenon of life,*
> *the gift of life, is so pleasurably serious.*

> ~ Boris Pasternak, *Dr. Zhivago*

I frequently considered the notion that I was being punished for trying to live. I am not sure to this day how much of that notion can be attributed to perception and how much of it rose from becoming more aware of the actions and motivations of others. I felt I was the target of relentless criticism from some of my closest associates.

The parish that I had supposedly controlled for nearly seventeen years began coming apart at the seams, thereby manifesting the words of the Psalmist, "When the Shepherd is stricken, the sheep will stray."

Throughout the period of my treatment and recovery my every gesture, word, nuance and action seemed to me to be under undue scrutiny. I felt a pervasive ongoing, and unnatural court of judgment forming among certain members of the congregation I had long trusted.

Looking back over the years of my ministry, I was struck by the number of individuals who had become empowered with the confidence I placed in their leadership capabilities. Sometimes the potential for leadership I thought I saw did not develop. More often I found that those I had helped groom for positions of leadership became emboldened by having achieved a position of influence within the community.

Antony Gabriel

Then too, some of the growing problems may have stemmed from the fact that the church and parish business were among the few avenues to some sort of status open to some members of the community. It was easy for me as the focal point and leader of a community to overlook the possibility that some are not always at ease with the power leadership grants, and cannot meet the challenge of wielding it gracefully. Perhaps, also, I expected too much of professionals and worldly and successful businessmen with good educations. One learns that education does not necessarily make a person kinder or better; nor is it a key to a winning personality, as I learned with some of the attending physicians. Education is but a refinement of natural talent that one uses, it is to be hoped, for the common good. Power in the hands of the spiritually dormant brings mischief in the same way it does with ungoverned children on the playground.

I tried hard to maintain a sense of humor concerning the politics in the community, drawing on the genes from my mother's forgiving nature and my father's "laissez-faire" attitude in the face of every adversity from which he managed to rebound. I wanted to maintain a perspective I could live with without feeling I'd capitulated. On the other hand there were stretches of time when I was in tremendous turmoil, feeling sensitive, raw, exposed. This was related in part to the barrage of chemicals in my system.

In the family, as well, the stress of a serious illness can create havoc, especially if there are unresolved conflicts or issues. An emotional earthquake shakes the formerly serene terrain and lesions are opened when a life is in the shadow of death. Once the after-shocks cease reverberating, both welcome and unwelcome memories are exhumed.

Never before had I known such tensions in the lives of our immediate and extended families as occurred in those difficult days. For me as the receptor, my role as father figure crisscrossed all the boundaries of my extended family in the parish. Looking back, it seems that my illness unleashed all the nascent "demons" lurking in the background of our life as a family.

I wanted my wife and children to know the real me, or at least the me I aspired to be. Even though I had thought I provided my wife and

GABRIEL'S DRAGON

children with a materially secure life, I had an awful awakening to the fact that David, Mark and Tammy, and subsequently their children, felt they really did not have much of me. They had had to share too much with others and with the demands of a large, busy parish.

I recalled the Biblical saying, "What shall it profit a man to gain the whole world and lose his soul?" I acquired prominence in the Church and community and, perhaps without seeing it, lost my children emotionally.

I had always been aware that they were all good kids, especially in an era of social experimentation and ultra liberalism. Lynn saw to their upbringing. We'd made the decision after a few months in Montreal that I would do whatever I needed to do to be an effective pastor, but Lynn and I *both* could not leave the children to their own devices while we busied ourselves with the heavy schedule of social events which are part of the community's natural fabric. If I was the priest of the parish, Lynn was the priest of our home. With three teenagers, we didn't want to increase the usual risk of temptation to youthful misadventures through a lack of parental supervision.

I asked myself exactly what was my attachment to these children who are not married. Our children remain children to us forever. I shuddered at the prospect of dying and having them look at my corpse while saying, "Bye, Dad, whoever you were!" I think they believed that everyone else was more important to me. I was Father Antony, Super Priest, *rotten father* ....

I became guilt ridden thinking of my beautiful, independent-minded daughter Tammy, who had married young and was now living in New York. I saw more of the boys, by now in their twenties, and still living in Montreal. They often joined us for breakfast or dinner. Mark, with his sparkling eyes and quick wit was able slide in some stinging observations in the cross-the-table banter that were a real eye-opener for me. Oh, God, I thought to myself, if I have failed at this, everything else is but ashes and dust. I have always felt very strongly that parents script their children for the rest of their lives; I was in absolute anguish! I began recalling scenes just prior to and during Mark's wedding which took place midway through my chemotherapy. He was the last to marry, and even though the wedding was happening at a time when we were

— 112 —

Antony Gabriel

experiencing incredible stress, we all wanted his celebration to be as special for him as it had been for his siblings. I did not want him to feel his celebration was worthy of anything less than our best effort. I threw myself, as best I could into the wedding preparations, as we all did. Lynn and I hosted family and friends who came to Montreal.

In recollecting I can see just when and how the chemicals took over. I remember obsessing over the fact that there would not be enough liquor for a party we were hosting at home and ordered several cases, despite the fact that the basement was already full of much more than enough of everything. I was out of control and went on a buying spree. In addition, I wanted to impress Mitzi's family with my social prowess; to show them we really knew how to entertain properly and how capable we were by throwing a huge bash for our children.

The week-end of the wedding, family and friends, including my mother, were seeing me for the first time since my battle with cancer began. It was simultaneously a pleasure and an ordeal. It was delightful to see everyone, but it was also a strain on my limited energy. Everyone seemed to have so many questions. It was too much!

True to his nature, Mark had been thoughtful in setting the date so that it fell after chemo week, but we didn't know at the time that the week after chemo would be equally miserable with my body still reeling from the chemical barrage.

When the last child marries, the parents realize that a certain threshold has been crossed. I wept during the ceremony until I felt Caitlin patting my hand, "It's OK, Poppy, Mark is fine," she reassured me.

I ended up leaving the reception early, exhausted and unable to maintain any sort of composure. I heard the party went on for hours … life goes on. Tammy's children, Janna 4, and Ryan 6, arrived home with Lynn before the others. They climbed on the bed and nuzzled on either side (for longer than I'd ever seen either of them be still), bringing with them a feeling of warmth beyond all expression.

Nick Haddad, from Chicago, a young man we considered a third son, also left the reception early to come by, and brought the comfort of his beautiful smile and the sweet reminder of his father, Larry, my dear friend who had died unexpectedly a few years earlier.

GABRIEL'S DRAGON

Our children are our eternity and hence their children are an extension of all our hopes and dreams. When I was finally alone, I could not escape the flood of sentiment which seemed to overwhelm me. Did I really do the best I could have for my children? I don't know how long I wrestled with the demons of guilt before I gave in to the weariness in my bones and was mercifully rescued by sleep.

> *Sweet are the uses of adversity*
> *Which like the toad, ugly and venomous*
> *Wears yet a precious jewel in his head;*
> *And this our life, exempt from public haunt,*
> *Finds tongues in trees, books in the running brooks*
> *Sermons in stones, and good in everything.*

> ~ William Shakespere

Ordinarily, I did not keep a diary. When I made trips to the Middle East or Russia, I maintained a journal of my travels that were later published in various church periodicals. This, however, had been a journey of a different sort. This was a pilgrimage inward about which I felt compelled to write.

This record-keeping process began as a way for me to regain and maintain mental clarity. So many things were happening and I wanted to keep track of my own emotions which seemed to change frequently and without warning. I wanted to lay the events bare for myself, to view them later in the rawness of the experience as I shed the outer layers of my soul. I hoped I would be able to use it later to try to make sense of what happened.

I was unable to continue my writing on history that I had undertaken for the Archdiocese because of my extreme difficulty in concentrating, but writing about what was deeply personal, scars and all, came quite easily. This method of reflection kept me focused and permitted introspection about the relationships that I had established over the years, the mutual flaws and virtues of intimacy.

I did manage to write one article during that time based on the diary

Antony Gabriel

I was keeping which was published in *The Word*, the official magazine of the Antiochian Church in North America. That article is currently distributed to patients in various oncology units in Montreal. I also wrote a poem (which appears unedited at the beginning of this book) which revealed to me the shattering of my own seeming invincibility.

> *The more a man enters the light of understanding, the more aware he is of his ignorance. And when the light reveals itself fully and unites with him and draws him into itself, so that he finds himself alone in a sea of light, then he is empty of all knowledge and immersed in absolute unknowing.*

> ~ Symeon the Theologian, *11th Century*

Throughout the strange and new (to me) incidents that unfolded as if on parade in my mind, a small voice kept insinuating its question over and over again, "What am I supposed to learn?"

At one point, Dr. Gruner, perceiving my torment suggested I join a therapy group for cancer patients, but I immediately rejected the idea. For me that seemed a horrible prospect! Part of my thoughts on that matter stemmed from the fact that I felt, as a priest and pastor, I needed to keep some part of myself to myself, and these wounds I was experiencing were far too sensitive, and in places too *private* to expose them to strangers. Furthermore, some cancer patients die ! I wasn't ready to cope with anyone else's tears and fears, I'd had plenty of that in the parish.

I later agreed to see Dr. John Pecknold, privately. Friend and psychiatrist, he was a great support in both capacities. For some years he had been head of psychiatry at St. Mary's Hospital. He is primarily in private practice and associated with the Douglas Hospital in Verdun, Quebec. John is also a practicing Catholic and active in his parish. He became my father confessor and spiritual guide, having a broad knowledge of the Masters, Eastern and Western, that shaped the religious tradition of Orthodoxy and Catholicism.

I owe a tremendous debt of gratitude to him for seeing me through some of the most tormented days of my life. He came often to my bedside and spoke to me frequently on the telephone, far and above the call of duty. I saw John weekly, sharing my cares, frustrations and anxieties with him. His wise counsel helped me stay focused, even in the darkest hour when I felt the wave of capitulation to the ravages of disease and treatment looming ... looming ....

John found the right words to strengthen and fortify me to help me resist caving in on myself or allowing my resolve to weaken. Even though there were days so utterly painful that I became nearly suicidal, he lifted me out of the black hole of depression.

We all know by now that foreign chemicals in the body have a way of altering and clouding one's thinking. They strike at the core of one's resilience. It seems to me that much more needs to be learned about the long term effects of chemotherapy on the body. We still do not properly understand how it plays havoc with one's reality, perceptions and coping mechanisms. The human will can be smashed to bits. Mine was frail and frayed; under massive assault chemically and burdened by the roles I'd chosen as Father, Priest, Teacher. It was my belief that I must never display human weakness. I recoiled at the very thought of frailty or defenselessness in my character or my body before I met John. He became my *staretz*[8] or elder in the truest sense of the word, helping to find my own way to a new perspective through which to view myself and others.

As a result of this process of intense self-analysis, under the guidance of a trained practitioner, himself deeply rooted in spirituality, I learned some poignant lessons. For example, friends and parishioners had always been able to appeal to my ego by telling me, "Only you can do this (or that) task or resolve this (or that) critical situation." I learned to recognize my own vulnerability and through that process acquired a new freedom. I had the right to say, "No, I am not the only one," or, "No, it is not my responsibility," or just plain, "NO."

NO. No wonder two-year-olds love to say that word! Ever notice the sense of entitlement they convey? They really believe they have the right to say no to anything they please. Can you imagine rediscovering that feeling after so many years of discipline and conditioning?

Another epiphany came when I learned that the old saying, "No one

Antony Gabriel

is indispensable," applied to me. Sure, things might be different, but life does and will continue to go on for me, the swashbuckler-twentieth-century priest. My emperor complex[9] was summarily flattened in the struggle.

How often have we heard the words, "Everything happens for a reason?" Well, there's a reason for that. There truly is no such thing as blind chance or fate. From the top of a mountain or the foot of a canyon; even on a boat in the middle of one of the Great Lakes with the shoreline nowhere in sight and in thousands of other ordinary ways, we are made aware what an infinitesimal part of the universe we are. The falsehood of one's self-importance is shattered by nature's immensity. The trick to uncovering the lie is to learn to notice.

Maybe for the first time, the true meaning of being centered struck me. Listening to the voice at my deepest center, brought a new passion for living. I began a new peregrination that lifted me above my former self, enabling me to better appreciate the majesty of God who is everywhere present, in joy as well as in tribulation. We have only to open our hearts to Him to receive lucid vision and ears that are more attuned to the sounds of silence. Thus our innermost Self begins the march towards transcendence. How else could one forgive the past and move forward in the present.

Even the Church itself took on a different texture in my mind. No longer was it a socio-political forum that propelled egos, but rather that locus for the internal evolution of the human spirit. The hollowness of institutionalism had been lost forever on my new horizon.

One day during a Parish Life Conference, a bishop asked me quite directly what I had learned most from my illness. Without any consideration, my instant response was, "Your Grace, I left the church for a while and drew close to God." Perplexed at this statement, he asked for an explanation. My answer had, I told him been simple, to the point and based on my view of the East's mystical intuition of what is the church. That was for me a manifestation of Fr. Jean Meyendorf's teaching that Jeus did not establish an organized religion but a mystical path for one to be *in-Godded.*

The Church as form and function, the Church as an external organization, the Church as posturing and programs, the Church as a

GABRIEL'S DRAGON

quasi-political forum where one receives self-affirmation; all these views disappeared with the advent of my new, clearer perspective.

The Church, for me had become what it was established to be: The beacon that lights the path.

I used to wax eloquent on this truth in sermons and written articles, without ever having realized that I had never internalized it. I knew it intellectually and even felt it at some level. Still, *The Church* was very much a concept; something, I served and was connected to. Today, as never before, I see the Church as a place to discover God and the God that is within each of us. It is no longer necessary to hold an office or position of authority, no matter how vital it might once have seemed, but only to grow in knowledge of God and His divine plan for us. Acquisition of the spirit is the one thing necessary. When it comes about we can work our own miracles, as the gospel promises.[10] What is the measure of a human being whom God has made "a little lower than the angels?" (Psalms 8:4). Humility, self-emptying, without which I am only an actor on the church's stage. The gratification of an actor, no matter how good the performance, or the show, is fleeting. After the bows, the applause ends, and what's left when there's no role to play?

It is certain that my candor startled my episcopal friend. One can never be whimsical about such a serious subject after having a life threatening disease and all that it brings in its wake. At Church conferences, it is not unusual to joke in small groups about the conditions of the Church, the world and society, either the confluence of interests or the lack of vitality. Such conversations are a favorite way for groups of clergy to deal with frustration.

In the after-hours coffee shop caucuses, there is much fixation of our society on the mundane, with its emphasis on competition and success, and how this has effected (and affected) church polity. In the western world, ecclesiastics on all levels are enticed by burgeoning numbers, large budgets, expanding building programs, complicated computer installations, and prideful proclamations or their leadership and prowess in these endeavors. So captivated is their concentration on these matters that the Spirit, is effaced, from the landscape by the

Antony Gabriel

capitulation to creeping secularism in the very organism created to foster immunity to that subtle disease.

Many of the Church Council members throughout the country boast to one another of their multifaceted technological advances, from vigil lights to church bells and sound systems. In some parishes, Church services are conducted synthetically through the use of tapes and digital discs! The church is, therefore, not exempted from the dilemma of having to deal with a society inundated with computer technology, professionalism and slogans and labels. In a word, modern man has chosen to view church growth as a phenomena lateral to, rather than, above and beyond societal norms.

One of heroes of early Christianity, Isaac the Syrian, indicated to his fellow pilgrims that "one who sees himself as he truly is, is even greater than the angels." He also pointed out that one must meditate on death daily while despairing not, only becoming more accountable for one's actions.

Someone once remarked that an insensitive soul exists as in a walking corpse. This is the meaning behind creative suffering. A crisis can lead a person to a deeper apprehension of the inner life and how our actions affect others, even those outside our immediate circle of relationships.

Everyday business creates shells around our hearts whereby we become mere functionaries who routinely perform daily duties and provide well in a material sense. All of this is nothing compared with the loss of quality of life or of life itself. Should life be construed to be the mere series of events and performances, or rather the glorious and perpetual simultaneous descent into the depth of existence and ascension to the summit of Being.

For five years prior to the onset of my illness, I had been teaching a course at McGill University entitled, "Eastern Orthodox Mysticism and Contemporary Literature." I found it to be illusive to some of the students, many of whom were simply looking for an elective, while a few were looking for something that would fill a void in their lives. Upon reflection, I believe I found it difficult to bridge this chasm because my course was not based on existential experience and deep understanding.

It was too intellectual. I taught it reasonably well, and even received praise from the majority of students, but I had not lived what I taught.

It was only during my struggle for life in the physical body and for the spiritual enlightenment, without which my soul would wither and dim, that I began to understand how all the pieces came together. I slowly began to appreciate in practice, the Eastern reality of the dignity of the human person, free will and the dazzling risk of communion with God. Claiming of the divine gifts that are waiting is a matter of focusing on the Divine. The crown among these gifts is bliss that we cannot even imagine and the jewel in the crown is that it grows and increases eternally ad infinitum.

Dag Hammarskjöld once said, "The longest journey is the one inward." There is no ascension without first plunging deep inside, to see oneself face to face, and there one can wondrously discover the face of God. Spiritual schizophrenia is overcome by just such an integrated thrust. The hard edges of the personality are softened and remolded by attuning the heart to the divine intelligence.

Biblical authors understood that it is within the heart that healing takes place. It is the locus of dragons and angels. The exorcism of one's inner demons is the first step on the road to recovery, to health. A fragmented, disintegrated, fractured mind impacts the body beyond any imagining and the reverse is also true. A fully integrated, whole person is well, radiant and at peace within and without.

Modern man, like his ancestors at the dawn of history, hungers and thirsts for the Other. We have constructed a panoply of "gods" but none can adequately quench the yearning for transcendence which happens when one struggles to reach for God.

It is true that we see the face of God when we love our fellow man, but the capacity, the wellspring of love is born from the wholeness which results from the union of the heart, mind, soul and spirit of the individual person.

The service celebrated on Holy Wednesday (the week before Easter) in the Orthodox Church is also a preparation of the Holy Oil used in the sacrament of Holy Unction for the healing of the infirm. During the

Antony Gabriel

Anointing Service all the consecration prayers for the holy oil appeal for the healing of the dichotomy between body and soul. In other words, the whole person must be engaged in the dynamics of the movement toward restoration, reconciliation and internal peace are two parts of one concept. As the Master said, "Thy faith has made thee whole. Go and sin no more." Behavior modification, (change, transformation, turning-around) is always a possibility.

My own personal life became, and continues to become transformed from the correct, external conduct of rites and rituals, form and function to that internal, intense leap into the heart of the Divine whose tender embrace brings warmth to the very core of our being. Agape and Eros burn together in a blaze of light that flashes inexplicably, momentarily, and ruptures the security of apathy and alienation. The incarnation of God in the flesh assumes and transfigures all passions and sensuality.

There is a marvelous ancient Syriac story about a young man who lay weeping by a brook. He began chanting in a sigh, this little hymn. "Would that someone pull me down and rebuild me, and make me a virgin again .... " In the stillness of the night, a sweet voice responded, " ... this request of yours is possible with the Lord." The gravitational pull of the Divine towards the center and as the center of all things, makes everything new again.

After a visit to the headquarters of the Archdiocese, the same bishop to whom I had spoken previously during the Parish Life Conference, inquired as to what I believed to be my most poignant thought during the entire previous year. My answer was, dread!

Taken aback, the bishop looked at me with a deeply furrowed brow and asked, "But you are a man of faith. How could you have experienced dread or been afraid of death?" I shrugged, smiled and side-stepped the question; a thing I would not do today. For some reason I was not yet ready to share with him my thoughts on the subject. Perhaps I felt that he, a celibate clergyman, with no real close ties to leave behind in death, could never understand my dread. I guessed, also, that the notion that one of his priests considered that death was a thing to dread was sacrilegious to him.

I never feared the dissolution of the flesh, rather it was the thought of separation from my loved ones that was the source of my dread. I wanted most fervently the experience of the roads we had yet to travel. As the cumulative effects of the chemicals in my body built up in my system, and I was overcome with weakness, premonitions of death swam around in the pool of my thoughts. In moments of steroid-induced surges of power, I felt invincible, but as those feelings ebbed, the prospect of leaving the world and being cut off from those I hold dear loomed.

In that period when I was sure I would be dragged into that dark tunnel, the sense was omnipresent. How could I be separated from people I loved so intensely? King David understood this when he wrote in the Psalms, "I looked at my right hand and there was no one there who would know me." (Psalms 142/141)

A person in this state is trapped in a state of agitated tension. On the one hand, intellectually and within one's heart, there can be submission and readiness to complete the journey. Yet, somehow, all the Biblical sayings and the promise of the kingdom often felt as much like a threat as a promise. The knowledge that one must be like a grain of wheat, and die in order to be reborn came to me as an illumination as I felt myself being drawn away.

On a purely human level, however, my resistance was rooted in a clinging to human affection and familiar surroundings that seemed secure. I knew for sure what was here on this plane. Like so many of those departing souls I had comforted, I too, feared the unknown and was humiliated by the fear because I thought I'd known! Waiting in ambush for me in the dark of many a night, the indescribable dread rippled just beneath the smooth surface of my serene and cozy surroundings.

Finally, I was grateful that the stuff of faith came to me through a yearning to be one with *The One* who is all. It was a beautiful, " … flight of the alone to the Alone … " the Infinite Friend. Much the same as in the dream I described earlier, I was touched by a moment of equally indescribable joy, the depth of which eclipsing, forever, the possibility that dread would ever again over-power my senses so completely.

Antony Gabriel

CHAPTER THIRTEEN

Picking Up the Pieces

Ignorance and sin are characteristic of isolated individuals.
Only in the unity of the Church do we find these defects
overcome. Man finds his true self in the Church alone: not in
the helplessness of spiritual isolation but in the strength of his
communion with his brothers and Savior.

~ Father Alexander Elchaninov, *20th Century*

In the summer of 1993 as I finished my course of treatment, there was also a series of conferences and conventions in the Antiochian Church Archdiocese. St. George Parish played host to the regional (Canadian/American) Parish Life Conference at the end of June. The organization and planning was carried out by the youth of the community under the guidance of my assistant, Father Peter. The Church's new Auxiliary Bishop, Basil Essey, presided and enthralled the participants by his humility and straightforward manner. I received many calls from conference participants, and on the last day, Bishop Basil paid a visit to me at home. He stayed only briefly since I was too weak to talk much. It meant a great deal to me that my colleagues had missed me during the conference and remembered me in prayer throughout the weekend.

Later in July, the national conclave took place in Pittsburgh, Pennsylvania. Having served the Archdiocese for over twenty-five years in several capacities, I was saddened not to be present. These conventions, for me, have always been like huge, holy, family reunions. Not only is Church business conducted, but people from all over North America unite around the Archbishop, and clergy and laity alike renew friendships every two years.

It was a strange feeling for a person like myself to have been absent from a major Church meeting. As I indicated earlier, I had at one time been certain I was indispensable. In this instance I recalled the business of the department of Credentials and Statistics which I have chaired for many years, and in which I had inaugurated many improvements, that I would have expected to dissolve into complete chaos without my leadership. By this time, however, I had learned that they would carry on without me. The pleasant surprise was that, where once I might have felt diminished by the fact that my important and difficult roles had been competently handled by others, I now felt relieved of a burden I was temporarily unable to carry.

As is always the case, my absence may have created a temporary vacuum, but it is never long before someone else steps in and takes charge. If we are fortunate enough to have been good stewards, we will have prepared the ground well for someone to do the work even better than we did. This does not imply that one is disposable as contemporary culture would have us believe, only replaceable. Each one's unique contribution to any institution abides forever, if it is unselfish.

There were some terrifically bright moments during the latter part of the year. A couple I knew socially, active members of the Jewish community, hosted a victory dinner party for me with my close friends in the parish to celebrate my return to active parish work.

Another time, Canadian artist Armen Tartousian (RCA) arrived at my home with a lovely painting as a thanksgiving offering for my

Antony Gabriel

recovery. My acquaintance with Armen was cursory, at best, yet he chose to do something quite magnificent.

Many of our friends both members and non-members of the church community sent contributions in my name to the various oncology units or caring groups at local hospitals. I was gratified to know that such awareness was raised through my travail. Other sensitive souls such as Yehouda Chaki, a world renown artist, was so moved by stories of my suffering that he reached out in the mist of the tender beginnings of our new friendship to give me much encouragement. Identifying with his own sense of abandonment during the Second World War and his exile spent in Greece, he shared my grief and elevated my soul by his creativity and humanity.

Such behavior illustrated the intimacy of the world we inhabit. No one knows the long term effects of their acts of kindness and generosity. It seems to me that this is what community is all about. It also added another dimension to the definition of family. We became a family of people, kindred spirits, helping one another by genuine and generous concern and seeking nothing in return. Ultimately, it is life itself that bestows us with grace upon grace, and a communion in community.

It is important for one who is on the receiving end of such wonderful deeds to acknowledge them. Much of the time I did not understand the full force of the impact a religious leader can have on those whose lives are touched by his ministry. For better or worse I had always charged forward as I saw fit but rarely, if ever, considering the ripple effect (again, for better or worse) of my approach to my work.

A few months later, Elias Abou-Shaheen, a friend who came to see me from Lebanon, purchased my ticket so I could travel to Detroit. Father George Shalhoub, a priest there, and Father Tom Ruffin, who had flown in from California, invited me to come for a brief but intense reunion. I had resisted their previous offers to visit me in Vermont or Montreal. While it was one thing to indulge my whims for companionship on a short term coming and going basis, it was quite another to consider the ongoing company of house guests. Besides, until this point, I could not have tolerated the invasion of my space by house-guests, even dear friends like these. I just wasn't ready.

GABRIEL'S DRAGON

Elias, a part-time Montreal resident, had his own reasons for choosing this time to visit and as the home he maintains in this city is near ours, he was able make almost daily visits during his stay that November. He told me with apologetic candor that he had been unable to bear the prospect of seeing me in some weakened state during the treatments so he waited until they were over with and I was well on the way to recovery. When he learned of the plans of our mutual friends for a reunion, he insisted I make the trip at his expense. He knew how highly I had valued the support of these two friends throughout my illness.

Fathers George and Tom, my closest allies and priestly soul-mates, had called me almost every evening to offer their love and encouragement. As a result, the bond between us is sealed forever. They hosted a dinner at that reunion gathering clergy friends from the Midwest. My friends seemed to be deeply touched as I painted a verbal picture of the cataclysmic events of my life over the past six months, and how I had managed to survive the ordeal. We spent a few joyful days together telling stories and making each other laugh, pastimes at which these two seasoned priests were more adept than most men.

One story concerned the call I had placed to Father George at his church during a late evening reception. It took place in the month of June during the crisis and hospitalization I described. I carried on for so long, not wanting to hang up, that he passed the phone around to all the guests most of whom didn't even know me. I remembered only that I was grasping at any straws available to affirm that I was still alive.

The meeting was highly charged emotionally. Our relationship goes back several decades, and it was the first time we had seen one another since I was stricken. I learned later from a former parishioner from Toledo, Ohio, that when her pastor, Father Michael Elias, preached that Sunday, he decided not to give his prepared sermon. He spoke instead about our meeting in Detroit, the stories we had shared and the manner in which my illness had impacted on our relationships.

Antony Gabriel

What is the thing we crave most in life? The sense that someone, somewhere remembers and loves us. Even better if we loved them in turn. Anything can be endured if that idea holds fast.

~ *Red Square*, Martin Cruz Smith

We celebrated American Thanksgiving in Vermont that year. Former Seminary classmates, Father Maximos Moses and Mark Campbell with his wife, Nettie, along with a former assistant, Steve Adams, flew in for the holiday. It is strange how an illness can impact on friends. There was a new, nearly palpable awareness of how fleeting life is. It becomes an imperative to demonstrate solidarity to those with whom there is a bond, as if the solidarity is some sort of talisman bringing invincibility. Perhaps, in many ways it is.

I was still behaving strangely and people walked on tiptoes to keep from ruffling my feathers. It turned out to be a very nice way to be thankful together, despite my uneven emotional state.

I returned home Saturday to attend the wedding of a couple to whom I had committed to be at least in attendance. Starting out from Vermont, I was very tired but as I crossed over to Canada, I felt the energy beginning to pulse through my veins. Listening to the soundtrack from "Sleepless in Seattle," I started singing along, gesticulating, and shouting, "I am alive! I am ALIVE!" Dusk was falling, I would be home soon; all was well.

Suddenly, a car stopped dead in front of me to avoid hitting a dog on the highway and I plowed into its rear. I smashed my hand and broke it on the windshield. I got out of the car and wept uncontrollably in disbelief of what had just happened. A passerby stopped to console me while her husband called the police on his cellular phone. I was taken to the hospital in St. Jean-sur-Richelieu and released with a temporary cast, into the care of my son Mark who had rushed to fetch me.

On Monday, Lenny Ayoub a friend drove me to St. Mary's Hospital where I could receive a proper cast. On the way home, I insisted we stop at the new store of Magid Tarabulsi, who had requested a blessing before opening for business. Getting out of the car in front of his shop, my foot caught in the long strap of the leather carrying case for my Holy Water sprinkler. I slipped and fell onto my back in a snow bank as the bag flew through the air. I lay on my back in the snow, as people passed on their way from office to home and I raised my fists to the heavens and shouted for all I was worth, "What are you trying to do with me? I have suffered enough! If you want to get rid of me, just do it, but stop torturing me. I thought we were a team! Stop, already! It's enough!" I dissolved into a combination of laughter and tears watching passers-by give me a wide berth as they hurried by what surely looked like a deranged man lying near their path.

Certainly, in some ways, I was quite deranged. Who can tell for sure which of my body cells still retained remnants of the chemical cocktail and when they would choose to stomp all over any good judgment. In addition, I had not yet comprehended how to put into practice many of the truths I had learned. I was still not listening as carefully to my body and its messages as was necessary for a true healing to come about. The chemicals were still in charge. Therefore, I continued, to do intermittent damage to myself from time to time and consequently to those who were closest to me. I realize now, of course, that I really should have given myself some real down time where I didn't marry, bury, baptize and officially bless but I had to prove, and keep on proving myself to myself, over and over for who knows what reason. I apologize now and forever to those who loved me most for the fear and anxiety I now know they suffered daily. My family truly expected on a daily basis to get a call to come and scrape me off of some floor or wall.

> *About suffering they were never wrong,*
> *The Old Masters*
>
> ~W.H. Auden, *Musé des Beaux Arts.*

The unusually bleak winter of 1994 was mercifully broken up by a trip to Chicago to celebrate the twenty-fifth anniversary of the parish there.

Former parishioners and friends traveled great distances for the dinner at the Union League Club of Chicago, arranged by Albert Joseph. We spent the entire evening relating tales of how we had organized the parish against all odds.

They wanted to see me and I wanted to see them. We had shared so much during the years when the parish was taking root. One former parishioner stood up at the conclusion of the festivities and said, "Thank you, Father Antony, humor and faith, laughter and commitment, joy and community. You knitted us together in the difficult period of structuring a parish in a major metropolitan area, and today you brought us together once again to celebrate something special. You are still very much a part of our lives."

Another young person stood up spontaneously and said, "I am here, because when I was young, you took the time to talk to me and make feel that I was an important person. You were the only one to guide me through troubled times. You listened and believed in me. You made a difference in my life."

I was made to feel that I wasn't just a former pastor but a friend and spiritual father. Letters, calls and little notes and expressions of affection, many from a great distance had a curative effect. I was told that quite often people were gathered in groups for prayers for my health.

The power of community prayer must never be underestimated; it is a mystical, synergistic bond that connects the faithful everywhere. I had been told that I was in the liturgical commemorations of scores of friends all over North America, the Middle East, and Russia. The daily mail brought bulletins, prayer cards and handwritten missives indicating that my name had been inscribed in the worship services and that intercessions were offered for my health.

There is much evidence of the power of prayer offered on our behalf. There is an invisible mystical presence that reveals itself in so many ways to one who is suffering. It is most often beyond the exterior comprehension of the beholder, but not beyond the person engaged in the agony of struggle for survival. Transcending time and space, the convergence of positive energy forces have an unspeakable influence on well-being. If one is receptive, the power of prayer embraces and nourishes our souls. I was told by Georgina that her young daughter said, "God was ready to take Father Antony, but we all protested and He accepted our plea to keep him with us." It occurred to me that the innocent prayers of the children and the pure supplications of the elderly, whose wisdom and forbearance I cherish, had been extraordinarily effective in energizing my battle.

At one of my lowest periods, the Eastern Orthodox Clergy Association of Quebec celebrated a liturgy for my recovery at one of the Montreal Greek parishes. It was a very moving experience initiated by Father George Saitanis. The priests surrounded me at the front of the large church, supporting me physically and spiritually. I sensed the collective energy that flowed from the praying brethren into me as I stood at the side of the altar. Although weakened in body, I was strengthened in spirit. At the close of the service they all embraced me, and at that moment, their gift of love was so tender and sustaining.

I found all these manifestations of support, love and encouragement incredible. Did I deserve such an outpouring of affection from so many quarters? An overwhelming sense of unworthiness befell me and again I counted myself fortunate to be so bountifully blessed.

That the blessings and prayers came from people of so many diverse religious and ethnic and social backgrounds was an affirmation that such affinities need not be exclusive but are, rather, inclusive and that the inclusiveness is another manifestation of the image of God in human-kind. Love and compassion (co-suffering) transcend the boundaries of the so-called religious. The cadence of faith, after all, opens the hearts of all people of good will. Somehow, I do not think there are denominations in the Kingdom which is (all) our Father's house.

As the new century loomed, the clearest message it brought was that if there is to be a survival of humanity as we know it, the reaffirmation of community is essential. If the last century was marked by the rise of individualism, the next century will see a redefinition of community. It is the sense of community and the universal knowledge that we still do

Antony Gabriel

need one another as parts of the body of the human family that will ultimately save this planet.

In this light, I was so deeply moved by loving acts outside my immediate circle by people who had absolutely nothing to gain by their outstretched hands and hearts. Relationships don't just happen. Lives intersect one another for a reason, and again, we flow in and out of one another's spheres when we least expect contact. To paraphrase St. Paul: "Neither height nor depth nor distance can separate us from the love of God," ... and one another. The world is indeed a very small place ....

> *All religion is the spirit of Love;*
> *all its gifts and graces of love;*
> *it has no breath, no life*
> *but the life of love.*

~ William Law, *17th Century*

CHAPTER FOURTEEN

New Beginnings and a Sabbatical

It is standard procedure throughout chemotherapy to have intimate contact with the primary surgeon and oncologist. Both doctors, Beliveau and Gruner, maintained a vigilant watch over me for close to two years. They supported and, at times, contradicted each other about the prospects for my recovery. Often, I needed some input from Lynn to help interpret their assessments; I heard what I wanted to hear depending on my mood at the time. When one of the doctors would be effusively positive, the other would cite statistics based on research and data that indicated the uncertainty of my plight. When I wanted to resume pipe-smoking to relax, one of them told me to, "Go ahead, you might as well enjoy the time you have left. It can't hurt you in your present state."

The period following treatment during the monitoring of my reaction to the chemotherapy can be summarized as a time of erratic emotional vacillation. I approached each appointment with either unfounded confidence or unreality-based fear with no apparent trigger for either emotion. I would march in for the office visit full of vigor only to stumble out deflated; or I would walk in with great trepidation and wind-up leaving feeling lighthearted, ready to click my heels and skip. I never knew which emotion to expect.

When I went for the surgeon's exam in August 1993, Dr. Beliveau told me I looked great and seemed all clear. Dr. Gruner told me in his office later that day that I was in remission. I went to church on Sunday and told the congregation my news. They stood to applaud.

When I returned a week later to the hospital for more blood tests, I was told not to be so quick to get my hope up for a quick recovery. I was told that once you get cancer, you always have it. They said I should remember to consider the statistics. They said they were being honest with me by telling me that colon cancer is an unpredictable disease, especially at my stage of the game. It was acknowledged that while I had, indeed responded quite nicely to the treatment, the protocol was still experimental and the full ramifications were not yet kown. Hearing that made me feel defiant! I determined that I would show them all that I was in charge of my body and nothing unknown was going to happen.

I was told that I had to be checked each month by the oncology unit, and every six months or so by the surgeon and I kept the commitment and did as directed until December 1994. At that check-up, Dr. Beliveau told me, "You have made my practice worthwhile; you are healed wonderfully on the inside, but remember, you are only in remission."

I made a decision after that visit not to be held hostage by the disease. There were no more signs of cancer at that time and I truly believed that there would be no more cancer! I also decided not to keep coming back for check-ups and tests as long as I felt good. On occasion when I saw my doctors in the corridors when I visited sick parishioners in the hospital they still conveyed a sense of astonishment in their looks. I had beaten the statistics. They plainly told me they expected a recurrence by a year or so later. Ten years later, it has not happened.

One of the main reasons I found it so difficult to keep up with the regular blood tests was that the pervasive odor of the oncology unit brought all too vividly the period I spent there undergoing chemotherapy. It might have been an easier task had the follow-up tests been scheduled in rooms other than the part of the hospital where the treatment was administered.

Today, as I continue to make hospital visits, I walk silently into the oncology units as a sacred place.

Later, I also asked to have the porto-cath removed. It was supposed to remain for five years in case of a recurrence. I felt somehow that it was negative conditioning to expect the worst, having learned that our subconscious rarely disappoints us. Furthermore, as long as that hard, uncomfortable lump remained in my chest, it would be a constant reminder of a difficult period, making it impossible to move past the whole period into another phase. Besides, it often became infected and was a constant source of irritation. I wanted it out, so out it came.

This does not mean that I advocate complete disregard of physician's advice. It is simply to say that a time comes when one must also be attentive to an inner sense of what is best in one's own individual situation for the promotion of physical and mental health. No life-threatening disease or situation encourages cliff climbers without adequate gear. There is no encouragement from this quarter to take needless risks.

Recently, Dr. Gruner convinced me to return for the normal blood tests at his office, and once again, the results were clean.

It was apparent to me, even though it may have been too soon for anyone else to recognize it, that I was a changed man. The chemicals still had a foothold. I was easily aware of the limits of my energy, but still not ready to give in to them so easily. The bottoms of my feet were full of deep cracks and my feet hurt which made walking difficult. It took many months for my taste buds to return and to begin to regain weight. My new hair finally started coming in blacker and thicker.

There were a few residual benefits to being a recovering patient. When you're back from near-death, people quickly return your calls, just in case. The adjective, courageous is hyphenated to your name. Your appointments can be expedited quickly or you can cancel at the last minute without fear of being considered rude. The weight and hair loss is usually marked enough for people to push you to the front of a waiting line, provided you remove your wig or hat.

That was all well and good, as were the newly rediscovered revelations concerning truth, beauty and the unity of mankind with the universe. On the very human level, despite the support of so many and

Antony Gabriel

the acknowledgments, which meant so much to me, I was becoming frayed in spirit and short-tempered. By this time, unlike when I had been immersed in the chemical fog, I had progressed to where I was aware of my snarliness. Evidently, along with some of the loftier qualities (mentioned earlier) that had been passed on to me by my father, I had inherited the impatient gene. I brooked little small talk and began finding large crowds oppressive. The official social side of my public ministry became increasingly irksome.

When I ventured out, on the better days I was acutely aware of how out-of-touch people seemed in their pursuit of trivia. The superficial chatter of cocktail parties so offended me that I could comfortably make only the briefest appearances. The endless questions about my condition became troublesome reminders that I was not yet quite whole, so to avoid that discomfort, I retreated inwardly, a necessity for my survival. How often I wanted to explode when people I barely knew posed intimate questions with smiling faces and what seemed to me a form of ghoulish curiosity. Although theoretically well fortified, I was not quite psychologically, emotionally or physically ready to deal with the real world.

I had reached the point where it was time to try pulling some sort of logic out of the mental blur and I was trying really hard. No simple task! I passed a large portion of my time in Vermont, and on some weekends returned to the city to preside over liturgy. There was constant contact with my church office by telephone.

It occurred to me that I was often being taken advantage of when I projected myself into the public arena. I had changed but no one else had. Part of the process was that I subjected every situation to intense scrutiny. Why was I present at this function? What was my purpose and how would this further its accomplishment? Time, effort and energy were all more precious than ever and thought was needed for their wise allocation. I became restless, feeling simultaneously positive and negative emotions which often translated into actions I see from today's perspective as having been self-destructive. Whenever I accepted an invitation, the avalanche of requests for more assistance in some area became an overwhelming burden.

GABRIEL'S DRAGON

I became so aware that I was overreacting far too often. For the benefit of all concerned, myself included, I stepped back a few paces for a while. I had traversed such a large terrain in my attempt to carry on life-affirming activities, that I had dissipated whatever resources I had. In order to live with cancer, I had barreled along until I came to a full stop with the realization that I was doing damage to myself, to my ministry and to my family. The entire illness and its aftermath became a watershed in the critical evaluation of a priestly ministry.

The restlessness which had surfaced just prior to my having been diagnosed now emerged in sharper focus. I had not allowed sufficient time to heal, just as my physicians had cautioned all along. They had written to church leaders insisting that I take a smaller role in the administration of the parish. All the professionals treating me felt that I was too involved in too many issues at once, on the personal level as well as in my work. It had even been suggested that I should consider retiring with the role of Pastor Emeritus.

After discussion on this subject, the parish council supported and assisted my taking a sabbatical for six months to retrieve my soul. I returned to Vermont. There I attempted to rechart my career and make decisions about my priestly vocation in Montreal and in general. Lynn had been hoping this would afford us more time together, but while we shared the same space, other preoccupations took hold of me.

During this sabbatical, which began in the summer of 1994, I threw myself into writing the book that had been in my head for many years. During that six month period, writing was a form of therapy. By immersing myself in the maze of manuscripts, letters and research documents late into the evening, the terrible ordeal I had just undergone gradually receded. Foremost in my mind was a feeling of urgency to leave a literary legacy that would prove useful to scholars and students interested in the development of an ethnic-Arab Church in North America in the twentieth century.

This work both elevated and exasperated me. I had to meet deadlines and re-examine thousands of documents. Finally, late one night, I pulled out all the stops and began working feverishly. I continued

Antony Gabriel

for many months until the project was completed. During this time I was asked to write an extensive article to commemorate our church's centennial celebration in 1995. This appeared in printed form and was distributed later that year at the Church's biennial conference in Atlanta, Georgia.[11]

It had taken me more than a year to regain sufficient strength and lucidity to write creatively. Some understood but others did not, that I had deadlines to meet. A large part of the credit goes to Georgina Howick and the team she put together to help me. Georgina shepherded and helped finance the project with others until the manuscript was sent to the Archdiocese for publication.

After the rush to complete the article, the book itself was nearly ready for submission for publication. In my research, I had unearthed many original letters and other documents buried away in archives and even old Arabic books. Many had to be translated from the Arabic, Russian, Greek and French sources. In the spring of 1995, I submitted the manuscript to St. Willibrords Press in the United States. Some ten years earlier I had promised to add a volume on the history of Orthodoxy in America to a series already published by that house. Although other publishers had expressed interest, I wanted St. Willibrord's to be the one to bring out *Ancient Church on New Shores: Antioch in North America.*[12]

The book was accepted and this success gave me the push I needed to write a second book, the one you are now reading. At the Church conference in Atlanta, after many hours of talking about my experience battling cancer and surviving chemotherapy, two physician friends encouraged me to either tape my experiences or write this book. As the history project, I sat at my desk in Vermont and started to write. I wrote both from memory and from my diary, and the words poured forth. In ten days of quiet in the mountains near Stowe, this book took shape.

One compulsion in writing a book such as this is the certainty that one will be able to refocus. When someone writes in a journal or diary, he can pour out his entire soul on the pages. Keeping a diary allows a person to take a step back, peer into the past and review the relevancy for today of previous commitments.

The past can offer a creative impetus for honorable deeds, or it can be a life-choking noose around the neck. There are images, shadows and figures that loom in our consciousness and sub-consciousness that need to be seen clearly and understood. In order to live freely, a person must appropriate what is positive and exorcise what is not.

While I am not a trained psychologist, I have lived and experienced enough of life to know how complex are the scripts we live by. This is one reason I cannot emphasize often enough the importance of forgiving the past when it hurts. An Arabic proverb says that, "He who has no past, has no present and certainly no future." A mature, integrated, balanced person has the capacity for harmonizing these elements without diminishing one at the expense of the other.

Later in the fall of 1994, during my sabbatical, I accepted an invitation by several Lebanese businessmen, former residents of Montreal to visit them in Lebanon. They had returned to resume their lives after the war ended and to help in the reconstruction of their country. Many of expressed their desire to visit me during my convalescence, but I had simply not been up to the effort. They understood my reasons and offered the trip to celebrate my recovery. It would also allow me to personally thank the president of Lebanon for having an award he had bestowed on me earlier that year the rank of Knight Commander of the Cedars of Lebanon for my work with the refugees during the height of the war.

In the early days of their immigration to Canada, the Lebanese businessmen in particular lived lives separate from their children. Many of them commended their youth to our care while they struggled to earn a livelihood in the Arab world. They knew of our work for the poor as well as our concern for their youth. Many of these young people accompanied me as I made my rounds of the parish, or came to our home for meals to fill in the blank spaces in their lives as teenagers in a foreign country. Their parents lobbied strenuously for official government recognition of my efforts upon their resettlement in Lebanon.

I was deeply touched by their generosity. Accompanying me were Fathers Tom and George. Inclusion in this experience was also my gift to them, a way of saying thanks for their continued friendship.

Antony Gabriel

Furthermore they did not want me to make this trip alone. Lynn, too, was somewhat ambivalent about my going. She worried about the stress of a long journey to the Middle East, with the climate and diet changes. My closest colleagues, therefore, arranged to leave their parishes in the fall to come with me.

I was also anxious to make this voyage as a pilgrimage to the Convent of the Presentation of Our Lady to acknowledge my debt of gratitude to my dear cousins, Mother MaryJo and Sister Balagia Tebshraeny for their intercessions on my behalf. I wanted to travel to Syria to the ancient Convent-Orphanage of Saydanaya where the miraculous Icon of the Virgin, reportedly written by St. Luke, is housed and there make an offering of thanksgiving. Both Christian and Muslim pilgrims travel vast distances to make vows or venerate the sacred relics at this sixth century bastion of Christian witness.

Our friends and sponsors as well spared no effort to make our two-week stay a feast of lights. We spent some precious time with the Patriarch of the Antiochian Church, His Beatitude, Ignatius IV, at the venerable St. Elias Monastery in Dhour Schweir. It was at this very spot that the 1966 voyage to Lebanon had taken such a dramatic turn. Since this was my first visit since the war in Lebanon began, it conjured many fond memories.

I felt like a celebrity with the attention from the media, the chauffeured limousines and the visits from so many who came to see me at the resort hotel where we were staying. The testimonies of appreciation from former parishioners was overwhelming and very touching. One such witness took place during an extravagant dinner reception. The food manager turned out to be a woman we had assisted, a Maronite Catholic who had come to St. George looking for a job. When she learned the banquet was in my honor, she stayed long enough to say a word of thanks.

Our stay in Lebanon was a humbling experience. That so many with no motivation other than to say thank you did so with such extravagance was quite moving. Sweet memories of those days passed in Lebanon will abide in my heart forever.

CHAPTER FIFTEEN

A Return to Reality

Who then devised the torment? Love.
Love is the unfamiliar Name
Behind the hands that wove
The intolerable shirt of flame
Which human power cannot remove.

We only live, only suspire
Consumed by either fire or fire.

~ T.S. Eliot, *Four Quartets, Little Gidding IV*

It didn't take long, however, for a major setback. Just when a person is flying high, believing he has the world by the tail, there is often a time bomb ticking in the background. While I was in Lebanon, Lynn phoned to tell me that a crisis had erupted in the parish. It was something that had been brewing since the onset of my illness. In the church temporal as in other (often unintended) political entities, when those next in command sense any weakness in the leadership they are emboldened by a new feeling of power and very much like foolish children in their reckless wielding of it. Being far away and not having all the facts, I had to sit tight until I got back. On the return flight to Montreal, even though I had just been elevated to new heights of enthusiasm, a wave of anxiety washed over me as I wondered what new dilemma awaited me.

Cold reality faced me as soon as I deplaned. My secretary of many years had clashed with my young inexperienced assistant. She had worked for me for fifteen years, as well as with great devotion for the entire parish. As a result of this confrontation and some poor judgment on the part of some of the council members, Nancy left her post, and I was plunged into a storm that shook the entire parish. It was no coincidence that this happened when I was out of the country. It was made very clear to me by those responsible that their own suspicions of improprieties in our relationship were cited as validation for their ending an extremely successful partnership. It had been a partnership that had worked well for the church and the community and even for the benefit of those who sought to destroy it. For the Gabriel household, Nancy was and continues to be a treasured member of the family.

In addition to this initial greeting on my first day home, the following events took place over the next two days:

On the domestic front, ceilings in the front bedroom and living room of our Montreal home had caved in leaving the second floor of that house in disarray for months. It seemed part of a never-ending saga of mishaps.

As if that weren't enough, while lunching with the Parish Council executives, I received a phone call from the Brossard (a community on Montreal's South Shore) police, who were looking for me. According to them a warrant had been filed with Interpol for my arrest. No matter that my name only happened not to be the same as that of the Iranian businessman who was wanted in connection with a crime; and no matter that I did not happen to fit the description of the man they were looking for, I could, I was told be arrested at any time. While these particulars were the most obvious of mistakes and seeming the easiest to resolve, it took months of effort in dealing with miles of red tape (because of a computer error) and a huge toll on my energy. I cannot begin to imagine what kind of legal fees I'd have had to pay without the intervention of some powerful voices on my behalf! I received only a cursory phone apology after the matter was cleared up!

Wondering (only fleetingly) if I was being punished for having enjoyed a moment in the sun, I felt zapped and sapped by the barrage of complex situations that had surfaced in rapid-fire succession upon my return.

Then came another curve. The insurance company which covered my medical expenses was taking legal action against me because of a technical error caused by a miscommunication during those confusing and fearful days just prior to my surgery. Add to that my astonished disheartenment at learning that the small coterie of council members, whom I'd been sure I could count on were the same ones who were harshly judgmental concerning any adverse situation in which I found myself.

"Heads up," my inner voice warned! Two sure lessons I'd learned from the past were about to be called on for the sake of caution and support. First lesson: If a leader shows any sort of weakness, the weakest and least loyal of the followers will swiftly and mercilessly find him disposable. Second lesson: The devil doesn't knock us off our feet by offering any delightful or overwhelming temptation. That would be too obvious. He simply and very subtly erodes our will until we capitulate. The devil seduces us by turning our attention to doing battle with the legions of small problems that keep us off balance. He revels in the minuscule clashes. All we can do is be true to ourselves. It is only love and humility that ultimately prevail.

Even with the inner red flags having gone up it was difficult to meet the challenge of defending myself against the onslaught that came from the most unexpected quarters.

As I mentioned earlier, our parish had been engaged in a costly building project. Now, since my illness, for the first time since beginning my pastorate in Montreal I was not leading the troops in raising funds for that project. This became one source of insecurity among that earlier mentioned small (increasingly vocal and negative) coterie.

Antony Gabriel

That week I returned and those that followed as I attempted to complete my history projects and gradually assume pastoral activities was marked by upheavals in every part of my life. It seemed that on a daily basis I was confronted by some new problem. And for no reason I could fathom the most intimate details of my life came under harsh scrutiny by those of whom I was counting on to hold the fort until I could get back to fighting strength.

Throughout the years, I had delegated the execution of many of my ideas to subordinates while standing in the center to keep the disparate parts of parish life and projects together. Being virtually absent for a year, once I took a break from standing at the center, the deep chasms on many levels at home and in the parish became evident.

Each week there was another explosive, soul-shattering crisis to be dealt with. The small group of council members would materialize in the office as self-appointed crisis managers which might have been fine had they really been doing their job and managing the crises! Their way of crisis management was to march in, define the crisis, as they saw it, then place the blame squarely at my feet before going out to beat the bushes for another mess. It was as if they were gathering evidence for a trial, but they had to work very hard to manufacture the crimes first and sought my cooperation in my own undoing.

My physicians, John Pecknold in particular, were concerned that this sort of continual bombardment would sabotage my recovery as each encounter with this group became a shock to my already frail psyche and health. While the overwhelming majority of our parish and the entire community remained enormously supportive, the inner core, or a small band became increasingly insensitive to my plight.

One explanation for the unsettling conditions was surely connected to the fact that that they did not want any blame or burden, for financial responsibilities in the parish (which was in fact their actual raison d'etre) in the face of the current sliding economic and political climate in the province. It is normal for insecurities to arise when any institution embarks on projects that place it in debt, such as we had taken on, during uncertain economic times. The political climate in Quebec, with

GABRIEL'S DRAGON

the continual talk of separation and sovereignty, and the lack of a countervailing voice, created deep anxieties among people who were immigrants or children of immigrants who had already at some point faced serious political instability in their lives. Businessmen who are ordinarily generous in their charitable donations find themselves tightening-up under such circumstances. Whoever is in charge, (the leader) then becomes the focal point for the expression of their frustrations and the dumping spot for blame or responsibility they seek to escape.

That small circle even spoke among themselves, and often in my presence, about the possibility that my illness had been greatly exaggerated or exploited to avoid work and to take financial advantage of a now financially overburdened congregation. Clearly, during the period of my sabbatical, there had been rampant insecurity and chaos had been given free reign.

This experience of a kind of subterrean opposition and attempt by a tiny minority to influence and level the church leadership (in this case *me*) under the guise of good stewardship is a recurring phenomenon throughout my historical study of The Church, as well as churches in general.

A common thread binds the eras together in my historical study of The Church. In the earliest period, the saints and martyrs had to contend with operatives of the state or the emperor who demanded obeisance to their gods. The Church was subsequently persecuted for its lack of fealty to this secular power because of its loyalty to another kingdom.

In the early part of the 20th Century in North America and abroad, the Christian Church had to deal with the topsy-turvy political systems in the Middle East as well as in the Eastern Bloc countries, hence the large-scale immigration of citizens from these countries to North American shores.

During our era, the secular has taken over as the twenty-first century loomed ahead. Believers, including clergy, face a new kind of persecution: psychological martyrdom. There is a self-service arrogance among secularists, some of whom, for various wordly reasons seek

Antony Gabriel

positions of lay-leadership within the Church. This posture proffers the illusory "truth" of its own assertion of rights. Pastors have an invisible but tangible adversary that decapitates authentic spirituality. This spirit maintains firmly, "It is the bottom line that matters."

One needs to be vigilant to avoid succumbing to this invisible power that wears many faces. Once an eclipse of the spirit occurs, a downward spiral begins. I found it terribly difficult to maintain my equilibrium in the face of these constant subtle and not so subtle challenges.

Daily negative forces have a way of imposing themselves and to distract by using the tools of depression or despair. The little droplets of despair falling relentlessly on our hearts and minds have as their goal to deplete the will so that the only alternative is to surrender. Whatever one accepts as the devil, there is never a need to look far for victims. It is generally accepted that one of his favorite playgrounds is the Church, where dissension among parishioners derails the positive initiatives towards God. One can readily notice tempers shortening in complicated church services. If a detail is omitted, a wrong tone chanted or a child misbehaves, the knowing congregant tsk, tsks.

I have found it equally true that the skilled tempter delights in our vulnerability to him through illness. He whispers in our ear, "There is no hope. Reject God. He did this to you. Give in. Give up." There is no mercy in the seduction of the spirit.

If a human soul gives ear to this seduction, it will surrender any capacity to plug into God's immense grace. If it is time to leave our earthly home and the soul does so bitterly while complaining about God's injustices, then hope is abandoned and reconciliation with God is never sought.

A human being under this evil influence can reject the love of family and friends, believing, often subconsciously, "Maybe if I anger them enough, push them far enough away, they won't miss me." The cycle of negativity overtakes a person who reasons thusly. Responding to the rejection, the patient wallows in self-pity saying, "No one truly loves me; no one cares," or, "I am being punished for my ugly persona, therefore, it's best to leave now."

In order to avoid this self-justifying cycle of negativity that feeds on itself, when any family member is hit with a life threatening illness, the whole family has to keep talking. We do not always comprehend how vital it is to talk, or that by not bringing things into the open we can rob each other of a unique opportunity for growth. Communication leads to openness and can have a positive impact on health and well being. We can best use this sacred time as an opportunity to pray together, to talk and to mend or deepen relationships.

I too discovered, as much through the anger and hurt expressed by my son David during the incident described earlier, as through several other examples, how significant the inability to communicate can be. Things left unsaid can leave a legacy of regrets. As a priest and pastor, I know that talking is most therapeutic. In the Eastern Church, confession is a Sacrament. It is a Sacrament of talking. When a person empties himself he can be filled with grace. If one stays in icy silence, how can he know the warmth of healing? It is no accident that we are a generation that seeks opportunities to talk with psychiatrists or reveal our innermost secrets via the airwaves to "sympathetic" talk-show hosts.

Whatever happened to religious discussion, family talk and genuine candor between friends? Whenever we spill our guts (the metaphor here is not coincidental) a certain restoration or healing process is set in motion. When we can freely articulate our feelings, we can more readily come to terms with the disease and seize control of it before the reverse happens. This abides also for any psychological pain one experiences in life. This long held truth was another rediscovered gem in my experience with John Pecknold. As my sickness and the subsequent demons it unleashed unfolded I needed help to re-establish communication with my loved ones.

The Semitic world throughout the ages has been revered for its gifts in the oral tradition of storytelling and the preservation of lore through the written word; hence the scriptures which have been cherished for generations. Carefully chosen words can do so much to reach the heart and soul of a person gazing into the unknown.

The human psyche has an inherent need for communion. Aloneness gestates narcissism and inwardness and self-absorbed depression. Talking helps one to understand that he is not alone; that he is not the only one on this path. Here, again, from a very personal point of view I refer to my own experience of feeling isolated and misunderstood during the onset of my illness and therapy, and to Dr. Gruner's recommendation that I join a therapy group. Certainly, each person is unique and it is difficult to truly understand the suffering of another, but if we are catalysts for real communion, we help the person see the disease in a different light. It need not be the awesome feat it may seem.

Throughout the years, I have availed myself of whatever means came to hand to help people struggling to unburden themselves; a long walk in the park; a conversation over coffee or tea; or sitting at the bedside clasping the person's hand in mine. Often this was sufficient catalyst to invite an outpouring of pent-up emotion, pain or long-buried feelings of guilt that blocked inner healing and therefore forgiveness.

> *You give but little when you give of your possessions,*
> *It is when you give of yourself that you truly give.*
> *There are those who give with joy,*
> *and that joy is their reward.*
>
> ~ Khalil Gibran, *The Prophet*

I continually sought out the sick and suffering believing I had a special mission to speak out and help vanquish their doubts and fear. While my doctors continued to caution me about becoming too involved or over identifying with patients, I knew better. Surely at times it can be depressing to keep talking about illness and coping with its pain. On the other hand, I gained courage and strength from the battles of others. In fact, I have received far more than I have given. Their blessings, and their heartfelt gratitude continues to sustain me beyond measure.

The Priest, Minister or Rabbi is often seen as a bogeyman, and his or her presence is seen as an admission of defeat. I have heard

GABRIEL'S DRAGON

parishioners say so often, "Don't go in there, you'll scare her. She'll think she's dying." How silly! This could deny the person the opportunity of undergoing real catharsis. Maybe the silent presence, or a Biblical passage, or prayer is the uplifting space the person needs in order to cope, to heal, to reconcile, perhaps to convey God's consoling word.

One who is really dying knows from within that this is so. There is the familiar small, still voice from within speaking truth in the language only that listener can understand. Why stifle the spiritual impulse that may be waiting to come to fruition? The person's finest hour may yet blossom in such moments. Companionship is a healing antidote.

There is a mysterious relationship between each person and God. Sometimes we transfer our own feelings of apprehension or a lack of faith, onto the suffering person who is the very one who needs God more than ever before. Who are we to say no for the one undergoing immense inner pain, let alone the physical struggle.

I have seen firsthand the need for communication, reconciliation and support. There was a period when I believed fervently that Lynn was the "Wicked Witch of the World" because of her aggressive approach to my well being. We finally worked it out but it took time, effort, in-depth conversations, in short, almost literally, blood, sweat and tears, on numerous occasions.

Clergy need training in dealing with parishioner-patients who have been given the speech letting them know they are gravely ill with little hope for recovery. Every gesture and expression from a religious leader is taken as a sign of something important as every nuance is scrutinized and interpreted. It is, therefore, always important that visiting clergy be aware of the weight his very presence carries for the person he sees in any stage of an illness. It is never enough to pop in and offer a formula prayer. A brief visit, because the people who are dealing with life-threatening diseases do not generally want their space interrupted, may give the person the comfort and support, or even the opening, that's needed. Small doses of tender time with each person are the best tonics. Asking a question such as, "Do you want to talk?" can lead to an outpouring of

Antony Gabriel

emotions that can be healing. The clergy in general need to be sensitive to those lying helpless whose life lines are tubes and medications. People who are suffering need the touch of humanity. This is just one more of the truths I rediscovered first-hand.

Having been in the hospital bed, I now have a different view of medical caregivers and communication. Their gestures, nuances and tones are, to the majority of the people in their care, part of the fabric with which they weave whatever mood that will permeate their being for many hours after the doctor had left the bedside. Words must be measured carefully and not allowed to spill out randomly. I have seen many miracles and unbelievable recoveries against seemingly insurmountable odds. On the other hand, I have seen people cry themselves to death because of the brutal way in which they were handled. An aloof physician can have a dramatic negative effect on someone reaching out for answers.

Medical people need to have the courage and take the time to speak with their patients and key family members; look them in the face, connect with their eyes, and, without giving false hope, at least try to ease the person into the awareness of the gravity of the illness without overwhelming with hard truths, facts or statistics. Yes, medicine-folk it is a fine line. Please walk it! I am not saying that doctors should take over the role of counseling or act as group therapists for the family. Those who choose to study the sciences available for the healing of their fellow man, can undo all their good work with an irritable inflection of voice. The most recent literature is full of information about "treating the whole person," a concept which is, of course, long overdue in the West. What I'm saying is that medical practitioners must go one step further and use the whole person to treat patients. The dignity of a person must be an equal part of the equation.

Often the team of attending physicians and interns march in and out of the room like storm troopers. Their continued presence is often intimidating, especially when they whisper things about the patient in his presence. I remember one instance where there was a group of doctors huddled, whispering just low enough for me to imagine that there might have been something amiss and just loud enough for the buzz to disturb my attempted escape from pain in sleep. Then there was the female doctor who seemed hesitant to check my body wound, I wound-up reassuring her that it was OK, and that even though I was a priest, I was entitled to the same body parts. Her embarrassment was embarrassing to me and made me feel anxious under the circumstances.

And God will wipe away every tear from their eyes.

~ Revelations 7:17

In October 1994, I attended the oncology unit's Oktoberfest. When the doctors saw me so fit and active they were delighted. Inebriated with my sense of well-being, I told them, "Thank you for the surgery and the chemicals, but I thank the nurses for their compassion." It was the nurses who were there with me during the darkest hours. I said this not with bitterness, but with the joy of one released; I wanted to convey a message of healing and gratitude.

It is right to acknowledge every good deed done on one's behalf. Even Our Lord spoke about the one who turned back to say thank you for His healing grace. On a purely human level there can be no substitute for the time and effort it takes to remember small personal kindnesses of life. We may not absolutely require these remembrances, but when they do come they energize and are small touches of grace that keep us going.

By being thankful to one another as brothers and sisters in the spirit, we are also giving thanks to God. It seems to me that as God's children the only thing that we can offer him is our gratitude for his beneficence. God cannot force us to love him. Nor can we add anything to his stature. The one thing we can be is grateful children.

As the winter of 1994-95 began, Lynn was in a serious car accident which forced her to leave her job as a journalist and to seek intensive therapy and medical attention. Our son, David received his doctorate

Antony Gabriel

and left for a fellowship at the Mayo Clinic in Rochester, Minnesota, Mark moved to Florida and with Tammy living in New York, Lynn and I were left living alone together for the first time in over thirty years.

At this time the only thing I knew for certain was that God had given me another opportunity to serve and I was not about to accede to these apparent complications. In my heart of hearts, I made a renewed commitment, and the last thing in my mind was to give in or give up. There were days when I wondered whether or not I should resign, but those to whom I turned for advice urged me to stand behind an earlier decision to seek a new contract with the parish and I did so.

Recovering from a severe illness had already thrust me across an major frontier, and doing anything less than my best would be a betrayal of my instinct to stay the course for the long run. Too many were depending on my ministry, especially since it had been recast in the crucible of suffering. This new dimension would give new insights to a life dedicated to service. Uppermost in my mind was the realization of the resiliency of the human spirit in the face of adversity, an insight that emerged as I wrote this book. The early pioneers had to overcome the most deplorable conditions to survive. I believed I was no exception and therefore could do no less than they by continuing.

A Prayer

*O Heavenly Father, Touch and penetrate
and shake and awaken the inmost depth
and centre of my soul, that all that is within me
may cry and call to you.
Strike the flinty rock of my heart
that the water of eternal life may spring up
in it. O Break open the gates of the
great deep in my soul, that your light
may shine in upon me, that I may enter
into your kingdom of light and love
and in your light see light.*

~William Law, *17th Century*

Antony Gabriel

CHAPTER SIXTEEN

Onward

Nothing is permanent except change. The eternal circle of suffering and joy. When the leaves turn green again and the flowers bloom and the fruit ripens, the sting of winter's cold is effaced from memory.

~ Naguib Mahfouz, *The Harafish*

It is now over ten years since the descent into hell began. Can anyone remain the same as before? Even my skin feels different. After undergoing a traumatic happening, regardless of its nature, a person radically changes. Things I used to take for granted have become precious, and much of what seemed important in my past life has become irrelevant to me.

I have been blessed. The treatment was effective and I have been further blessed with more opportunity to serve in God's name, to have more time with my family and to set future goals. Still, each day remains a new challenge to reclaim my existence. Truthfully, no one can set a time limit to the physical or emotional limit into one's being.

Another truth that has emerged is that no physician can predict or be sure about every aspect of any catastrophic disease. I still experience considerable pain, internal discomfort and nausea. I continue to experience feelings of having been sawed in half, and no day or night passes without the sensation of persistent gnawing pain, which for many months I simply buried to avoid facing my own frailty. That was one of the behaviors which helped me into the mess in the first place!

The long terms of physical and psychological side effects of chemotherapy are not, in my view totally known or knowable. It's often said that (technically) the chemicals have been absorbed, metabolized, excreted, etc., by such and such a time. However, every cell in our body has its own memory! Doctors and researchers can never be sure or fully aware of the exact consequences, or the effects of one chemical on another vis-à-vis each individual body. In the final analysis, even though we are all thankful for interventions on our behalf from time to time, no one knows the body as well as the one who wears it. Any experimental program is just that. Experimental! Furthermore, any surgery or illness creates its own inner dynamics.

One of the residual effects on one who has confronted life and death through protracted illness and suffering, is that every issue is more quickly defined and categorized. I do not have adequate command of the language to properly describe the keen sense of clarity that comes to one who knows his life is about to be extinguished.

I must admit that this new gift has been like a daily wrestling partner. When interacting with others, it is very difficult to know the truth of a situation and still keep silent. At the same time it must be done very often to spare the feelings of someone who maintains an outrageous posture. Transparency is an awful burden when one looks through the facade of superficiality.

I no longer look forward to savoring the battle of verbal dueling that was once part and parcel of my interaction with the parish and its many organizations. I want to cut through the nonsense and tell people when I believe they are playing games. But how can I say anything and still allow the others to save face, especially, when I used to enjoy those same games?

On the other hand, the lushness of nature's colors seem brighter

Antony Gabriel

than ever before, and it seems especially so in the mountains which fill our view from the bedroom window in Vermont. It is a visual feast! I find deep contentment sitting on the balcony, looking around me and relishing the color and quiet.

I find large crowds de-energizing, so I prefer small groups wherein lies the possibility for the exchange of ideas to take place. I notice when invited to gatherings that people often want me to share some experiences from the period when I was ill and in treatment. Certainly it is cathartic to be so open about illness, particularly among Middle Easterners, who often view such topics of open discussion as taboo, and we have broken some barriers in this respect. The opposite is, however, also quite true. A person needs to move on in life and not continually define himself as any sort of victim, whether it is of illness or other life experience. Once the threshold has been crossed it is important to think of one's self as a survivor and turn the page to be ready for life's next adventure.

> *Sickness and health, prosperity and*
> *adversity, bless and pacify such a*
> *soul in the same degree. As it turns*
> *everything to God, so everything*
> *becomes divine to it. For he that*
> *seeks God in everything is sure to find*
> *God in everything.*
>
> ~ William Law, *17th Century*

CHAPTER SEVENTEEN

End Point, Beginning Point

The distance of several years has put much of the past in a proper perspective, although if I want to tap into them, those days are as fresh in my mind's eye as is this moment. Perhaps there is even more clarity today because there is more lucidity. I am simultaneously the same person I always was and a very different one as well, a point I try to drive home to my critics.

For years I thought that anyone afflicted with cancer or any other life threatening disease was like a prisoner, jailed in his own body, never knowing when the execution would take place. I find that this truth is a riveting reality. Most books on cancer testify to the haunting shadows of the disease, no matter how long one has been in remission.

While my realization of mortality flows like an undercurrent, I have learned that one can appropriate any experience into something creative. While there was a time when I enjoyed talking about myself, my suffering, my dilemma, I found it really difficult to maintain balanced relationships with others unless I shifted the focus from myself and moved on. Why keep boring others, who cannot totally appreciate the shock of the experience, even though they say they do? What difference does it make to anything? How much better it is to move on with life than to stay stuck in the past! It's today that counts. Yesterday is no more and cannot be changed or repeated, and the future cannot be controlled.

Every critical situation in life presents another opportunity for transformation. The will must be stretched to the limit; as well as the gravitational pull towards refocusing priorities. The elevation of the human spirit can occur when one makes the decision not to be defeated. In short, in the little victories of daily existence, one can reach beyond one's self with a hand outstretched to the other.

In helping others stricken with terrible illness, I have been blessed, endowed with a humble mission to share with others a way of dealing with all kinds of cataclysmic personal events. In these kinds of relationships, one appreciates the cross gifted to be carried and is grateful for those that lighten our burdens by walking side-by-side with us to Golgotha, as latter-day incarnations of Simon the Cyrene, who accompanied Jesus on the final part of his final journey, carrying the cross in his stead.

Suffering is, in fact, a special grace that carries the seeds of our transformation. In selflessness is transcendence. One must learn to let go of the past, to forgive past hurts and offenses, and put daily living in perspective with its setbacks and joys. There is a message in creative suffering that can expand one's humanity far beyond what was imaginable. One's horizon is enlarged by the unfolding. Suffering is an epiphany of the true person. If one is a barren wasteland spiritually, then suffering is a dead end. On the other hand, it can bear within itself the seeds for a fruitful harvest from the God-store that is waiting to be opened.

I would like to close with a story that illustrates the difficulty of wrenching words from the heart. It concerns Father Alexander Schememann, one of my professors and Dean of St. Vladimir's Theological Seminary until his death on December 13, 1983. His special area of expertise was Church History and Liturgy. In addition, throughout the span of his life in North America, he gained world wide acclaim for his broadcasts to the Soviet Union on Radio Liberty. Alexander Solzhenitsyn was among his many faithful disciples.

Father Alexander was by nature outgoing and witty. His intelligent lectures were always peppered with humorous anecdotes about Orthodox characters and world events. Educated in Europe, he was an extremely literate and articulate scholar whose interests covered a wide range of subjects.

His wife, Juliana, recently told me that on the day that Father Alexander learned he had lung cancer (which quickly spread to his brain), he noted the prognosis in his daily diary and then stopped writing. When he picked up the pen for his last entry, he wrote, "I have not written in my diary for the last nine months, not because I have nothing to say ... but because I did not want to fall down from the heights to which the sickness had lifted me ... *Lord, it is good to be here!*"

> *Our mind is pure and simple. When it is emptied of thought, it enters the pure and simple light of God, and finds nothing but the light.*
>
> ~ Symeon, The Theologian, *949-1022*

> *Be at peace with God, and many will come to find peace near you*
>
> ~ St. Seraphim of Sarov, *19th Century*

Reclining on the deck of our Vermont home, looking out at the many verdant shades of foliage and the pristine blue sky surrounding Mount Mansfield, I can only rejoice in this gift of sharing my life with others in the prayer of giving hope.

I have no illusions as to my future prospects. I have learned not only to live one day at a time, but one hour at a time and to appreciate every joyous moment of light. As one who has slowly and painfully emerged from the cocoon of illness and recovery, I know I must cast off any remaining gloom in order to return to take up life again.

Antony Gabriel

Does anyone know what will be hurled at us on the morrow? No one is exempted from suffering of one sort or another. It can strike like lightening. There are simply no assurances of what tomorrow will bring.

We must take advantage today, because the next moment is unknown. God has made no promises to us except to be there in the midst of our lives. We are not robots. We have free will. In that freedom, we have the ultimate gift of saying yea or nay to Him. The one thing God will not do is force us to love Him. This would violate the gift of freedom in humanity.

It is love that gives us the capacity to bear all things. Khalil Gibran wisely wrote in his famous book *The Prophet*: "Do not say that I have God in my heart, but rather, I am in the heart of God." This is the alpha and omega of life, unconditional surrender: "Abba Father." ~ Mark 14:36

There are miles to go before I sleep.

~ Robert Frost

Now I know only in part;
then I will know fully,
even as I have been fully known.
And now faith, hope and love abide,
these three; and the greatest of these is Love.

~ I Cor. 13:12-13

Prayer Of The Acceptance Of God's Will[13]

O Lord, I know not what to ask of Thee. Thou alone knowest what are my true needs. Thou lovest me more than I myself know how to love. Help me to seek my real needs which are concealed from me. I dare not ask either a cross or a consolation. I can only wait on Thee. My heart is open to Thee. Visit and help me, for Thy great mercy's sake. Strike and heal me, cast me down and raise me up. I worship in silence Thy holy will and Thine inscrutable ways. I offer myself as a sacrifice to Thee. I put all my trust in Thee. I have no other desire than to fulfill Thy will. Teach me how to pray. Pray Thou Thyself in me.

~ Metropolitan Philaret of Moscow,
19th Century

Antony Gabriel

EPLIOGUE

In the Lion's Den

As this book readied its completion more high drama was about to unfold in my life. Lynn and I had to cope with the loss of both of our fathers within a six week period. Death does not loose its sting no matter what age it strikes. The fact that both men died from cancer was particularly difficult for me to face.

During this period of mourning, I came to the unhappy realization that I would be obliged to reconcile myself to the erosion of the high standards of service that had been set for the parish community. My assistant left for the United States to start his first full time assignment. Much to my dismay, neither the associates who volunteered to help nor I could cope with the overwhelming pastoral demands during this turbulent period.

The most important commodity in a sprawling complex parish such as St. George's is knowledge; knowledge of the key players as well as all the family connections. In an ethnic Orthodox parish, the multiplicity of personalities necessitates that the best services afforded to the faithful of the parish requires insight into the sensibilities of each person. On a practical level, for example, when illness erupts in a family, the response must be swift, the caller identified and often, immediate action taken.

During that first year I confronted many crisis situations and extinguished many fires caused because my associates and the volunteers who came to my assistance, did not know the parish as I did. The pastor of an ethnic parish is by necessity a community leader and is therefore seen to be both public property and resolver of crises. This leads, quite naturally, to a steady stream of endless demands.

While it took another six months or so to manifest, there were smoldering fires ready to burst into huge conflagrations among certain of the parishioners. It seemed as though I was never far from the hot seat, in spite of its not having been through any fault of my own.

The last act of the story unfolds in a rather dramatic way and might properly be the subject of an interesting sociological study on the behavior of communities centering around religious institutions.

Since I had changed so much within myself during my illness, those around me had difficulty in either recognizing and accepting, or even realizing, that my agenda had altered profoundly. As I began to look more like my old self, people took advantage of my seeming well being to vent their spleens whenever the opportunity presented itself. My new softer persona was mistaken for weakness.

As an example of an ethnic parish in a highly secularized society, St George's congregation embodies the contradictions of a hierarchical church in a democratic milieu. The responsibility of leadership in such a situation carries with it similar paradoxes in both the religious and political spheres. The flip side of power, authority and authenticity is accountability, vulnerability and the full range of perceptions and projections of an often needy constituency.

When I was told in the late spring that continuing in the direction I was headed would end in a heap in some emergency room, I submitted my resignation to the Archbishop. At the same time I informed the Parish Council and the congregation that I planned to leave.

A few weeks later, during Great Lent, the auxiliary, Bishop Antoun arrived for a pastoral visit. He immediately sensed the tension within the parish – the stalwarts who simply refused to let me go and those who were in favor, for whatever reason, of my stepping aside.

Preparations were set in motion for a parish dinner in tribute to

Antony Gabriel

twenty years of ministry with a substantial burse from the parish. I began researching all availability of benefits for which I could possibly be eligible.

During Holy Week, emotions finally peaked. The entire parish seemed to come together in what proved to be the finest week of prayer and spirituality we had ever known. Young and old alone were pressing me to remain at my post while at the same time, the other faction was actively seeking my successor.

On the heels of Holy Week, I traveled to meet with the Archbishop to discuss my retirement plans. Succinctly put, he was adamant that I not leave Montreal. The reasons he presented were based on his knowledge and experience with early retirees who became ill after leaving active parish service. He also cited a host of reasons for my remaining: the double complexity of St. George's itself and the Quebec linguistic political dilemma coupled with the difficulty of selecting an adequate successor. Following several days of intense discussions which culminated in his agreement to send an assistant pastor who would shoulder the day-to-day responsibilities, I agreed to remain at my post.

Knowing parishioners and the Parish Council were awaiting my return from New York and the news concerning the future. Unbeknownst to me there were multiple caucuses related to my ministry in Montreal. Once I announced that the Archbishop had refused my request, and was sending an assistant to help, all hell broke loose. Many and varied interpretations concerning my short-lived retirement and subsequent reinstatement were circulating throughout the community. Once again, the saga of the past re-emerged in bold relief, and partisans from both camps expressed the full range of emotions. For some, it was a cataclysmic event in the closed world of the parish.

I discovered that the angst I had been experiencing over feelings in the parish had its foundation in actual events. My imagination hadn't distorted the situation. A rippling of discontent among former close associates as its impetus, was working to effectively stymie any plans I had for the parish. During that period I thought often of the words of my patron Saint, Antony of Egypt who cautioned, "We are tempted under the cloud of adversity until our last breath."

GABRIEL'S DRAGON

Once again, it was the women of the church who came to the rescue and organized a tribute in celebration of my twenty years in Montreal. Knowing my aversion to speeches, a musical and poetical tribute was organized with 700 people in attendance on a Thursday evening.

Despite my having offered to take a salary cut to assist the parish in the transition stage before the new assistant arrived, those in opposition wanted the event cancelled; however, for me and for many, it was a chance to encourage healing. I began meeting with the dissidents to discuss the reason for their resistance. I felt that face-to-face encounters carried more weight than either phoning or writing. However unpleasant it was to do a verbal striptease, I wanted everyone who had a problem with their pastor to state it, and move on. My physicians finally cautioned me against continuing that practice, warning that it would certainly have an adverse effect on my health.

As of this writing, an harmonious atmosphere has basically returned to St. George's with the occasional skirmish erupting from time to time to keep me on my toes.

The manifold interpretations of this period gave me pause. Internally I did not want my thirty-five year priesthood and twenty-year stewardship at St. George's to be a legacy clouded with controversy. This figured in my decision to weather the storm no matter the consequences for me mentally or physically. I felt it was in the best interest of both my family and spiritual charges that I stay the course and put the parish back on track. The road was not an easy one but one that needed to be taken.

Once again Mother Teresa's "courage" rang like a china bell in my head. I felt I had waged a successful battle with cancer and now I was called upon to wage another sort of battle with different disease. I thought about Daniel in the Lion's Den. The easiest road would have been to retreat; the more difficult one was to stay, face and fight the lions of opposition with the strength of faith.

Under the Soviet system, there were the so-called "wreckers" who disrupted Church processionals and liturgies as a cruel mockery to faith and ritual. There are coincidental occurrences in Western society by those whose particular psychological bent impels them to frustrate

Antony Gabriel

things being built by others for fear of revealing of one's own lassitude. Virtue, goodness and creativity can be an offense to any group not particularly touched by the grace of the Church. Therefore, the battle continues for anyone who has accepted to help bear "the Cross."

The perfect comparison of a person engaged in both the Church and the World is of one trying to empty the ocean with a sieve. It is an endless most thankless task. What sustained me were the faithful with their knowing wide-eyed glances. During that year, I encountered partisans who gave voice to a variety of concerns and special interests. I needed to dive headlong into each mindset to comprehend motivation and intention at every turn.

On the other hand, while it was more than evident that there was solid support for the direction in which the church was moving, detours were being simultaneously constructed to create confusion at every turn. It was gradually sorted out but it took my sudden resignation to the Archbishop, a reaction within the parish, and a solution for more pastoral assistance with a celebratory event of our 20-year ministry in Montreal to bring all the loose threads together.[14]

> " ... but this one thing I do: forgetting what lies
> behind and straining forward to what lies ahead."

~St. Paul to the Phillippians 3:13

On a philosophical note, one might look at Hegel's thesis, antithesis and synthesis for an intellectual counterpoint of what occurred in my church. On a spiritual level one might observe (as one leading layman confided to me that he had) that my illness, treatment and very uneven recovery were mirrored in the life of the Church. The ministry was so highly personalized that each impacted the other. Psychologically speaking, the interaction was such that no aspect was exempted from the trauma of the past three years. The ups and downs of the pastor as well as the unsettling conditions in Quebec produced a rash of meetings and counter meetings that articulated both rational and irrational expectations.

In the final analysis, I am even more firmly convinced that one must possess a solid vision of life in order to sustain a steady course. The psalmist says, "Unless the Lord builds the house those that labor, labor in vain." (Psalm 127).

The ultimate test of a person resides in the will; the inclination to willingly persevere in all circumstances and to strive toward the good. Redemption lies in the "overcoming." One must become what Nietzsche calls "Overman." It is the only response, the only answer to a series of obstacles placed in the way of anyone who has placed him or herself in the service of God and man.

It should also be noted that the modus operandi cannot be in response to barriers only, but there must be perpetual renewal within the community that elevates the consciousness of the active participants that the servants of God forge ahead daily. Each Dawn carries with it the hope and dreams for the new day of the Lord. Thankfully for this gift that the story has a happy ending. After several tumultuous years we all learned something about ourselves and hopefully are better for this experience.

It is my deep belief that while we are mere scraps, each one carries within a piece of the stars.

"My beloved speaks and says to me:
Arise, my love, my fair one,
and come away;
for now the winter is past,
the rain is over and gone.

The flowrs appear on the earth;
and the time of singing has come,
and the voice of the turtledove
is heard in our land."

~ song of Solomon 1 V. 10-12

Antony Gabriel

I Was Asked
to Write a Sketch

I was asked to write a brief sketch on the why of this book for the Cedar Cancer Institute's Board. It is difficult to write about one's own book; however there were several motivations that were compelling: namely, it was a catharthis and at the same time, a way in which I could translate a personal trauma in writing to help others who are likewise affected, especially by cancer.

This priest has *let it all hang out* for all to see, warts and all, in the confrontation with metatastic cancer. And for that matter, any life-crisis which threatens to knock one off his/her dime. It was special to chronicle my journey and to identify with the *Every Man* who undergoes dark days and nights.

Through the writing and publication of this book, it has been a persistent dream to be able to give hope and courage and for the sufferers to never give up or give in until one's last breath. As a wounded healer, it was gifted to this person to share experiences that would or could lead to a new spirituality that is life-giving. This personal account is also for the families to help them understand better in order to share the burden as sensitive caregivers.

Finally, each one of us experiences a variety of ups and downs in life. One of the great lessons that I learned throughout this period was that a priest must first be a human being and then a pastor. Secondly, is the largeness and capacity for forgiveness and letting go of persons and events to grow more completely in the peace of God. And this too, is for the Every Man.

I thank the Cedar Cancer Institute's Board of Trustees for their support for allowing me to share my life and thoughts. I prayfully hope that this little book will be a creative vehicle for Can/Support and beyond ... to help others.

Antony Gabriel

Message from the Publisher

Gabriel's Dragon Gabriel's Dragon! What a tremendous book to publish. It's as if, within the manuscript, came leftover trials and tribulations from Father Gabriel's previous ten years with the writing of this book.

When I think back over the prior sixteen months, it has not been an easy road for either author or the people at Abbeyfield Publishers to tread. Dogged by one problem after another, including the near death of Lynn, the author's wife, from a mysterious malady healed only just in time, and the computer and other disruptions caused to our designer, Karen Petherick, it seemed to me that the book was cursed in a way I could not fathom.

It was only when the book arrived to proofread in what I hoped would be the final phase, that I could sense a change in attitude ready to occur.

Editing can be quite stressful, sometimes a joyless occasion when one loves the career he has chosen in the literary field. But this time I stepped to one side and spent an hour or so meditating over what I held in my lap and its possibility as an inspirational book to others. I returned to it, took a deep breath, felt less stressed, and turned the cover of the manuscript to the first page. I began to read slowly and deliberately, concentrating hard to make it mean more to me.

Noise from my open windows subsided as I began to feel a better connection to the book. When I reached the torment of the man and the psychological eruptions and revelations he went through, his words began to touch my spirituality and I felt drawn closer.

Hours later, when I took a breather before finishing the last twenty-five pages, I felt I had cleansed myself of weeks of feeling offside. It was hardly Paul's conversion on the road to Damascus, but it was revealing, even calming. I'll stop my message on that word. Thinking of it and saying it aloud keeps me in my spiritual arena.

Bill Belfontaine
Publisher

Antony Gabriel

1   Page 1. Eastern Orthodoxy throughout the world is united in faith but organized geographically and according to the ancient patriarchal sees. Antioch is the third in prominence, but according to tradition, the oldest, having been founded by Sts. Peter and Paul. "And they were first called Christians in Antioch" (Acts 11:26) The Church in North America is part of the Antiochian Patriarchate.

2   Page 21. Dr. Edward Tabah O.C., also of Lebanese heritage, was one of Canada's premier cancer physicians and one of the founders and prime movers behind the Cedar's Cancer Fund at the Royal Victoria Hospital in Montreal until his untimely death from cancer in March 2001.

3   Page 29. This enabled me to receive the degree of Master of Divinity from St. Vladimir's Academy in New York. Later I completed the course and thesis requirements towards a Master's degree in Sacred Theology from LSTC in Syriac and Greek studies. For five years I studied and translated under the world-renowned Syrianologist, the late Arthur Vööbus. Under his tutelage, I gained the accredation to lecture at Oxford and later to teach at McGill University in Montreal.

4.   Page 70. In recent conversations with my doctors, I realized that they too had not been aware of these possible side effects. After my experience, they began to check in the medical literature. One article, "Canadians set Interferon Guidelines," by Pat Rich, appeared in the *Medical Post* on March 29, 1994.

5   Page 105. "O Lord Jesus Christ, the Son of God, have mercy on me, a sinner." This prayer is commonly used by monastics and pious pilgrims of the Eastern Church.

6   Page 107. See suggestions for further reading at the end of this book.

7   Page 110. Anna Awad Sopp's family distinguished itself as high ranking clerics in the Maronite Catholic Church in Lebanon, and Nazleh Tibshraeny Gabriel came from an influential family in Zahle, Lebanon, where her father held the title of "Shaikh" among the Orthodox Christians.

8   Page 116. In the Russian ascetical tradition, a novice inevitably attaches himself to an experienced orler monk, commonly known as a staretz.

9   Page 117. I recall now that at the height of my folly, I sardonically paraphrased Napoleon and Louis XIV saying, "The Church is me. I am the Church," in reference to all the success achieved at St. George during our 75th anniversary celebrations.

10   Page 118. Quote Jesus, "all these and even greater things, etc."

11   Page 137. It was published as part of the work entitled *North America: A Retrospective-Antiochian Orthodoxy in North America; the First One Hundred Years*.

12   Page 137. The Book: *Ancient Church on New Shores: Antioch in North America* was released in 1995. A second edition is in preparation to be published under the auspices of the Archdiocese by Antakya Press.

13   Page 160. A plaque donated to the Oncology Unit at St. Mary's with this prayer. I felt it would be helpful for those waiting for treatment to have a prayer which, I hoped, might ease them into a state of readiness for what was ahead.

14   Page 165. As of this publication: The projects have been completed with the restoration of the Church's interior decorated by the famous Emmanuel Briffa, with grants from the Federal and Provincial governments. Heritage Canada designated St. George as a national historic site in 1999. This, in addition to the reconstruction of the church's exterior and the construction of L'Habition St. George, independent appartments for senior citizens — adjacent to the Church with underground parking.

Appleton, George. *The Oxford Book of Prayer.*

Bloesch, Donald G. *The Struggle of Prayer.*

Bradshaw, John. *Creating Love.*
Healing the Shame That Binds You.

Canfield, Jack and
Hansen, Mark Victor. *Chicken Soup for the Soul.*

Chopra, Deepak. *Perfect Health.*

Cloud, Henry. *Changes that Heal.*

Cousins, Norman. *The Healing Heart.*

Dyer, Wayne W. *Pulling Your Own Strings.*

Emerson, James G. *Suffering: Its Meaning and Ministry.*

Fromm, Erich. *The Art of Loving.*

Gibran, Khalil. *The Prophet*

Goettmann, Alphonse *Prayer of Jesus/Prayer of the Heart.*
and Rachel.

Keen, Sam. *The Passionate Life.*

Killinger, Barbara. *Workaholics.*

Kushner, Harold S. *When Bad Things Happen to Good People.*

Levine, Stephen. *Who Dies.*

Lewis, C.S. *Miracles. The Problem of Pain*

Lloyd-Jones, D. Martyn. *Spiritual Depression*

Louth, Andrew. *Discerning the Mystery.*

Louth, Andrew. *The Wilderness of God.*

MacNeil, John J. *Taking a Chance on God.*
Mitchell, Stephen. *The Enlightened Heart.*
  The Enlightened Mind.

Moore, Thomas. *Care of the Soul.*
  Soul Mates.

Moss, Richard. *How Shall I Live.*
Moyers, Bill. *Healing and the Mind.*
Nouwen, Henri J. *Life of the Beloved.*
  The Living Reminder.
  The Wounded Healer.

Peale, Norman Vincent. *Positive Thinking Every Day.*
Peck, M. Scott. *The People of the Lie.*
  The Different Drum.
   The Road Less Travelled.
  A World Waiting to Be Born.

Peterson, Eugene H. *The Contemplative Pastor*
Samra, Carl. *The Joyful Christ.*
  The Healing Power of Humour.

Schutz, Roger. *This Day Belongs to God.*
Siegel, Bernie S. *Love Medicine and Miracles.*
  Peace Love and Healing.

Tournier, Paul. *Guilt and Grace.*
  The Meaning of Persons.

Vanauken, Sheldon. *A Severe Mercy.*
Ware, Kallistos. *The Orthodox Way.*
Warren, Samuel J. *Self-realization and Self-defeat.*
Wilkes, Paul. *In Mysterious Ways.*
  The Way of A Pilgrim. R.M. French, trans.
  A Book of Daily Meditations for Men.

Touchstones: *Night Light: A Book of Nightime Meditations.*
  Hazelden Meditations
  Series.

Antony Gabriel